SCHOOL HEALTH EDUCATION TO PREVENT AIDS AND STD

A Package For Curricular Planners

INTERNATIONAL ENCYCLOPAEDIA OF AIDS - 11

SCHOOL HEALTH EDUCATION TO PREVENT AIDS AND STD

A Package for Curricular Planners

Editor

Dr. Digumarti Bhaskara Rao

M.Sc., M.A., M.A., M.Ed., Ph.D.
R.V.R. College of Education
Guntur - 522 006
Andhra Pradesh (India)

DPH

DISCOVERY PUBLISHING HOUSE PVT. LTD.
NEW DELHI-110 002

First Published - 2000
Reprinted - 2015

ISBN: 978-81-7141-533-5

School Health Education to Prevent AIDS and STD

Published by:
DISCOVERY PUBLISHING HOUSE PVT. LTD.
4383/4B, Ansari Road, Darya Ganj
New Delhi-110 002 (India)
Phone: +91-11-23279245, 23253475, 43596065
E-mail: discoverypublishinghouse@gmail.com
sales@discoverypublishinggroup.com
web: www.discoverypublishinggroup.com

Printed at:
Infinity Imaging Systems
Delhi

Preface

The HIV/AIDS is a new phenomenon in the human society. HIV destroys the immune system of human individuals, producing a defenselessness fatal state known as AIDS. The World Health Organisation has estimated that already one in every two hundred and fifty adults in the world is infected with Human Immunodeficiency Virus and according to WHO's projections a total of forty million men women and children worldwide will have been infected with HIV by the turn of this twentieth century. Visualising the devastating effects of the HIV/AIDS epidemic within our life times and beyond is difficult. Probably, no other disease in recent times has had the impact on human society generated by HIV/AIDS.

The HIV/AIDS epidemic has brought into focus many health related ethical, legal and human rights issues. This epidemic requires immediate and effective responses in new programming areas: attitudinal and behavioural changes, community-based care and support initiatives, and the maintenance of human development in the face of increasing rates of illness and deaths. At this point, education enters the scene as it can alter the HIV/AIDS situation since it brings change in the behaviour of the people.

This *International Encyclopaedia of AIDS* presents the worldwide information about HIV/AIDS, issues and challenges, reports and reviews, ethics laws and human rights, and educational activities and programmes to keep the policy makers, planners, professionals, activists, researchers, educationists, teachers and students well informed of the epidemic.

Dr. Digumarti Bhaskara Rao
26 January 1999
The Republic Day of India

Acknowledgement

I am thankful to the World Health Organisation and its associated offices for using their material namely School Health Education to prevent AIDS and STD: A Resource Package for Curriculum Planners-Handbook for Curriculum Planners. Student's Activities, Teachers' Guide, Global Programme on AIDS-HIV Prevention and Care: Teaching Modules for Nurses and Midwives, Global Programme on AIDS. Community HIV Prevention Handbook; STD care Management-workbooks 1-7, Facing the Challenge of HIV/AIDS STDs: A Gender-based Response; HIV/AIDS and STD surveillance Data Management and Use-Report, Bangkok, 1995; Carrying out HIV Sentinal Surveillance-A Guide for Programme Managers, AIDS Prevention and Care in the workplace: Enhancing the Role of Private Sector; HIV Testing Policies and Guidelines; Carrying out HIV Sentinel surveillance; AIDS Prevention; Understanding and Living with AIDS; AIDS: A Modern Epidemic; HIV/AIDS in South-East Asia: IXth meeting of the National Programme Managers, New Delhi, 1993; Information, Education and Communication: A Guide for AIDS Programme Managers, Handbook on AIDS Home Care; HIV/AIDS in South-East Asia: A Pictorial summary; etc.

I am thankful to the United Nations Development Programme, UNDP's HIV and Development Programme, and UNDP's Regional Projects on HIV and Development for using their material namely Economic Implications of AIDS in Asia; Socio Economic Implications of the Epidemic; NGOs Working with Sex workers; NGO Responses to HIV/AIDS in Asia-Case Studies; HIV in the Workplace: Dealing with the Issues-Role Plays, Development and the HIV Epidemic, Law Ethics and HIV; HIV Law and Law Reform; Issue Papers; Study Papers; Working Papers; etc.

I am thankful to the Health and Nutrition Centre, Republic of Philippines for using its material namely sourcebook on HIV/AIDS Prevention Education for Tertiary Educational Institutions.

I am thankful to the Curriculum Development Programme, Ministry of Education, Government of Thailand for using its material namely Institutional Modules for AIDS Education.

I am thankful to US Department of Health and Human Services: Whitman-Walker Clinic, Inc., USA; East-West Centre, USA; National AIDS Control Organisation, Government of India; Academy of Culture Communication Education Science and Service, Guntur, United Nations and its agencies for using their material.

I am grateful to Bhaskar Bhattacharji; V. Alexeev, Geeta Sethi, Elizabeth Reid, Mina Mauerstein-Bail, A. A. Trinidad, Palomi Cuchi, D. Pushpa Latha for their kind co-operation.

Dr. Digumarti Bhaskara Rao,
Secretary
ACCESS
D-43, S.V. N. Colony,
Guntur-522 006

Contents

PART-I

Curriculum Planners

A

Designing the Programme

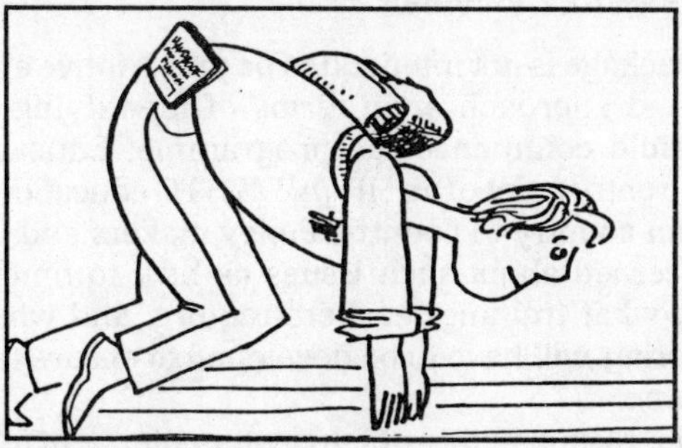

INTRODUCTION

There is increasing consensus about the need for AIDS education for young people. Studies have shown that sex and AIDS education may lead to a delay in the onset of sexual activity, and to the use of safer sex practices among those students who are sexually active. However, curriculum planners often lack examples of curricula, classroom activities and learning materials. This resource package has been compiled to assist curriculum planners to design HIV/AIDS/STD education programmes for their own school systems, for students aged between 12 and 16. The programme presented in this package is based on participatory methods, as these have been shown to be particularly effective for the teaching of behavioural skills.

The package includes:

• ***Handbook for curriculum planners***

Outlines the main steps in curriculum planning, and includes a series of appendices, mostly evaluation instruments.

• ***Students' activities***

Includes fifty-three student activities that meet a wide range of objectives for teaching an HIV/AIDS/STD programme. Curriculum planners may choose those most relevant to their country, and adapt the text and the illustrations for language and content, according to the cultural context and the age of students targeted.

• ***Teachers' guide***

Contains specific instruction on how to teach each activity, and background information for teaching a programme on HIV/AIDS/STD. This guide may also be adapted for language, content, and teaching methods.

Using the resource package

The package is not intended to be prescriptive either in terms of content and approach or in terms of identifying at what age students should commence the programme. Educational policy regarding the entry point of an HIV/AIDS/STD education programme will vary from country to country. Policy makers and planners will also be concerned about such issues as how to timetable such a programme, what training teachers require, and what additional printed materials will have to be developed to ensure the success of the programme.

It is the responsibility of curriculum planners to design their programmes. Their choices will undoubtedly be influenced by prevailing cultural norms and social and ethical values. Cultural, religious and ethnic norms and values must be taken into account when designing and introducing an HIV/ AIDS/STD education programme which deals with sensitive issues such as sexuality and safe sex practices.

However, it is also important not to lose sight of the fact that young people, for a variety of reasons, tend to adopt the norms, values and attitudes of their peers, which may be in conflict with those of their parents and traditional society.

Creating a collective responsibility

The Curriculum Planner has the task of designing convincing and effective programmes for students which will be acceptable not only to students but also to their parents and the wider community.

Students obtain all kinds of information outside the school and are often involved in experiences which may never be discussed or even acknowledged in a school setting. Care should be taken when designing an AIDS programme, to avoid discrepancies between 'school knowledge' and 'outside knowledge', as these can become a source of mistrust and conflict.

In this respect, it is important that the knowledge and skills acquired by students at schools, are sufficiently detailed and explicit to enable students to cope successfully with the situations of risk they are likely to encounter inside and outside school, including peer pressure.

The purpose of HIV/AIDS/STD education programmes is to provide students with the knowledge and skills which will enable them to behave in a responsible way and thereby protect their own health and wellbeing. Methods which will assist them in this respect, therefore, form the major content of this resource package.

Because of the sensitivity of some of the subject matter, it is advisable to involve families, religious organizations and other social organizations in the initial planning sessions. In this way, content and activities considered suitable for general classroom use can be identified, as can those which are considered necessary, but too sensitive for ordinary classroom teaching. Alternative methods for ensuring that the students receive the latter kind of information can be discussed and developed with parental and community involvement.

Community involvement contributes to a sense of collective responsibility and provides support, both of which are necessary if school HIV/AIDS/STD education programmes are to be successful.

Student involvement in the curriculum design process

When designing educational programmes, curriculum planners frequently include students in the initial discussions in order to ensure that the material will be relevant and therefore effective. Students have often been involved in discussions about social, cultural, sporting and recreational or community-based programmes for schools.

These discussions usually take the form of focus group discussions dealing with specific issues. Certain of these require a creative brainstorming approach. Focus group discussions can be held with many and varied groups of students from rural and urban centres and from various social groupings. In other instances planners prefer to work with a highly representative student group with whom they meet regularly and build up a strong and frank rapport.

Behaviour change and behaviour shaping are central to AIDS education. The behaviours concerned are highly individual and intimate and it is, therefore, crucial to seek the opinions and suggestions of students themselves about programme content.

Appropriate context for HIV/AIDS/STD education

The ideas and activities presented in the package focus specifically on activities related to AIDS. However, AIDS cannot be isolated from a whole range of problems such as use of alcohol and other drugs, early prostitution, teenage pregnancies, poor living conditions, violence, and unemployment. In fact, many of the skills and attitudes that young people need to prevent infection with HIV/STD, are life skills that will be useful in responding effectively to a variety of other problems that they may face as they grow up.

In particular, an educational programme dealing with STD, HIV and AIDS requires that students have an understanding of their own physical and emotional development during adolescence, so that they can gain insight into their own and others' sexuality. It is important to remember that the main mode of transmission of HIV/AIDS is through sexual intercourse, with the danger of infection greatly increased by the presence of an STD. Students should already have acquired basic knowledge about menstruation, sexual intercourse, conception, pregnancy and contraception.

HIV/AIDS/STD education is best taught as a component of health education, sex education or family life education programmes.[1] In those countries where such programmes do not exist, basic information about sexuality will have to be part of the HIV/AIDS/STD education programme.

PROGRAMME MODEL

Many programmes for the prevention of AIDS and other STD focus only on biomedical information such as the virus that causes AIDS, the immune system, signs and symptoms of AIDS, treatment. It is now well known that this type of knowledge is not enough to convince young people to adopt positive, healthy behaviours that prevent HIV/AIDS/STD. They need the motivation to act and the skills to translate knowledge into practice.

Infection with HIV and STD occurs in specific risk situations or scenarios: a girl is pressured into having sex with her boyfriend or an older man; a syringe with drugs is offered to a friend; friends pressure a boy to join them for a night out with bar girls. Young people in these situations need to have knowledge and skills to make healthy responses... how to say "no", how to propose alternatives, how to evaluate risks. If they receive only information on the immune system in their AIDS course, they will be poorly prepared to deal with real-life situations. Remember:

"The goal of AIDS/STD education is to promote behaviour that prevents the transmission of HIV/STD" and not merely to increase knowledge about AIDS.

A programme on HIV/AIDS/STD should increase knowledge, develop skills, promote positive and responsible attitudes, and provide motivational supports.

---

1 *School Health Education to Prevent AIDS and STD, pages 23-24. Comprehensive School Health Education, pages 3-5 and 10-12.*

• *Knowledge*

Information that will help students decide what behaviours are healthy and responsible includes: ways HIV/STD are transmitted and not transmitted; the long asymptomatic period of HIV; personal vulnerability to HIV/STD; means of protection from HIV/STD; sources of help, if needed; and how to care for people in the family who have AIDS.

• *Skill development*

The skills relevant to HIV/AIDS preventive behaviours are: self-awareness; decision making; assertiveness to resist pressure to use drugs or to have sex; negotiation skills to ensure safer sex; and practical skills for effective condom use. These skills are best taught through rehearsal or role-play of real-life situations that might put young people at risk for HIV/STD.

• *Attitudes*

Attitudes derive from beliefs, feelings and values. HIV/AIDS/STD education should promote: positive attitudes towards delaying sex; personal responsibility; condoms as a means of protection; confronting prejudice; being supportive, tolerant and compassionate towards people with HIV and AIDS; and sensible attitudes about drug use, multiple partners and violent and abusive relationships.

• *Motivational supports*

Even a well-informed and skilled person needs to be motivated to initiate and maintain safe practices. A realistic perception of the student's own risk and of the benefits of adopting preventive behaviour is closely related to motivation. Peer reinforcement and support for healthy actions is crucial, as peer norms are powerful motivators of young people's behaviour. Programmes that use peer leaders are effective because peers are likely to be more familiar with youth language and culture. Parents and family members can also motivate and reinforce the objectives of the programme and should be encouraged to play a part in their child's sexuality education.

Remembering that responsible behaviour is the key to prevention, the following 11 objectives are considered as a minimal requirement for any effective programme on HIV/AIDS/STD.

At the end of the programme, students will be able to:

1. Differentiate between HIV, AIDS, STD
2. Identify ways in which HIV can be transmitted
3. Identify ways in which HIV/STD are not transmitted

4. Rank methods of HIV/STD prevention for effectiveness
5. Identify sources of help in the community
6. Discuss reasons for delaying sexual intercourse
7. Respond assertively to pressures for sexual intercourse
8. Discuss reasons and methods for having protected sex if/ when sexually active
9. Respond assertively to pressures for unprotected sex
10. Identify ways of showing compassion and solidarity towards people with HIV/ AIDS
11. Care for people with AIDS in the family and community.

The programme units

The programme proposed in this package consists of four units, for which a number of classroom activities (with related teacher guides for each activity) are offered. The units are designed for different levels of knowledge, attitude, skill and motivation development.

UNIT 1- BASIC KNOWLEDGE OF HIV/AIDS/STD

The major emphasis in this unit is on: what are HIV, AIDS, and STD; transmission; protection; and sources of help. Approximately 25% of the total classroom time should be devoted to this unit. The unit covers objectives 1 to 5.

UNIT 2 - RESPONSIBLE BEHAVIOUR: DELAYING SEX

Students, particularly at early ages, should be encouraged not to have sexual intercourse. Delaying sex to an older age usually results in more mature decisions about contraception and protected sex. Students need to discuss the reasons for delaying sexual intercourse, and learn how to resist pressures for unwanted sex. Assertive communication skills should be learned through role-play of real-life situations that young people may encounter. They may also learn that affection can be shown in ways other than sexual intercourse. Objectives 6 and 7 are covered in this unit.

UNIT 3 - RESPONSIBLE BEHAVIOUR: PROTECTED SEX

Some, perhaps many students may already be sexually active at the time they learn about AIDS in this programme. Others will need to know how to protect themselves in the future, when they will be sexually active. Using a condom every time one has sexual intercourse is a very effective way to avoid infection with HIV/STD. Teaching students about contraception and condoms does not mean encouraging them to have sex; young people are exposed to information about condoms through a variety of sources (friends, media, condoms displayed in shops, etc.), and need to have information and skills on how to use them correctly. Objectives 8 and 9 are covered in this unit.

Units 2 and 3 on responsible behaviour should take approximately 50% of the total classroom time given to the HIV/ AIDS/ STD programme. This is because these two units are mostly concerned with developing skills, and this takes up more classroom time than learning facts.

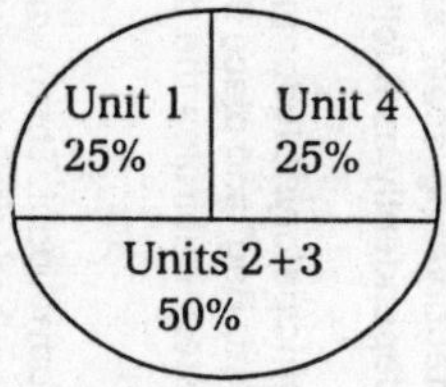

UNIT 4 - CARE AND SUPPORT FOR PEOPLE WITH HIV/AIDS

Many young people will come in contact with people with HIV and AIDS, perhaps in their own family or community. They need to learn tolerance, compassion and ways to care for and support them. Planners need to remember that people with AIDS may spend time in the hospital for treatment of acute conditions, but they are likely to live at home most of the time. Unit 4 covers objectives 10 and 11 and should take approximately 25% of the total classroom time allotted for the programme.

For each unit, a number of student activities are proposed. Curriculum planners will select those most relevant, and adapt them to local requirements. Here is an overview of the activities proposed.

UNIT 1—BASIC KNOWLEDGE ON HIV/AIDS/STD

Activity	*Rationale*	*Description*
1. HIV/AIDS/STD basic questions and answers	Basic information about HIV/AIDS/STD is essential to understand other concepts of the programme.	Informational (illustrated). A number of young people ask questions about HIV/AIDS/STD. The answers are given in "bubble" blocks.
2. Looking into AIDS	A pre-test to determine student knowledge is useful to both students and teachers.	Participatory. A short true-false test with a categoryating scale at the end. Can stand independently as a follow-up to Activity I .
3. HIV/AIDS/STD What do they mean?	Students learn definitions best when they can relate personally to the situation. A personal story illustrating the definitions is an effective learning tool.	Participatory. Students take definitions from "Grab Bag" and place them in the correct box. A story illustrates the definitions.
4. How a person gets HIV	Information on how the AIDS virus (HIV) is transmitted is essential to protection.	Informational. Three ways of acquiring HIV are described; the information is well illustrated.
5. You can't get AIDS by...	As well as knowing how HIV is transmitted, it is important to know how it is not acquired. This reduces irrational fears about the disease.	Informational with some participation. Students are asked to identify pictures of how HIV is not transmitted.

6. **What do you believe?**	This short test is an effective way of learning about the spread and non-spread of HIV, and provides rapid feedback to the students.	Participatory. A true-false test of 20 questions allows students to test their knowledge on transmisslon.
7. **What would you do?**	Stories about people's lifestyles, their risk of HIV and what they can do to prevent the spread, is an effective way to make risk situations realistic.	Participatory. Three stories followed by questions and a risk continuum encourage students to look at transmission from a realistic perspective.
8. **What is your risk?**	Students become more familiar with risk behaviours by classifying them as No Risk; Low Risk; High Risk. They also need to evaluate their personal level of susceptibility based on their own risk behaviours.	Participatory. Students evaluate 16 different behaviours and classify them as No Risk; Low Risk, High Risk. They also assess their own vulnerability on a scale of I to 10.
9. **Are you at risk?**	Similar to activity 8 but adds the element of multiple risk behaviours.	Participatory (small groups). Part I is similar activity 8 but involves 36 different behaviours per group). Part 2 portrays four different life styles each with multiple risk behaviours that are rated from highest risk to lowest risk. Part 3 asks, students to assess their personal vulnerability to HIV/AIDS/STD.
10. **Protect yourself against AIDS**	Students need to learn about specific means of protection.	Informational. Outlines four methods of protection from HIV/AIDS/STD in a visual presentation.
11. **Dear Doctor Sue**	Doctors are effective agents for conveying information about protection because of their	Participatory. Three letters involving protection; presented Students use the "Doctor's Bag"

Activity	*Rationale*	*Description*
	high credibility with young people. Dear Dr. Sue letters are motivational devices for conveying this information.	to get help in answering the letters.
12. Which is safer?	Students need to know the different ways of protecting themselves but they also need to know that some methods are better than others.	Participatory. Six patterns of sexual behaviour; presented and students are asked to rank them from most safe to least safe. They are to list problems with the methods that might cause a person to HIV.
13. What happens with HIV infection?	Students learn: the window period; time from infection to AIDS; AIDS to death; signs and symptoms; and infectivity.	Informational (graphically with illustration Outlines signs and symptoms and progression HIV to death.
14. How do you know if you have HIV/AIDS?	It is important to know that a person with HIV: - may have no signs or symptoms for a long time - can infect others during this time - gradually gets sicker and sicker and eventually dies.	Participatory. Involves three stories of people with HIV and/or AIDS. Asks specific questions about each story.
15. Testing for HIV	Basic information with regard to testing is needed by some students.	Informational. A student asks a doctor basic questions on testing. A "bubble" illustration is used to give the questions and receive the answers.

16. Test: what you know about testing	To recall information and understand concepts about testing, a "matching" test is provided.	Participatory. A matching test of 10 items and a category rating scale for correct answers help students understand concepts of testing.
17. AIDS help Who? Where?	Information on help sources for HIV/AIDS/STD is essential to this programme. Some students develop AFRAIDS (Acute Fear Regarding AIDS) and need help or counselling.	Participatory. Four different situations are presented through short case studies. Students are asked what type of help is needed and where they might find that in their community.
18. You be the doctor	Information about the following topics is important: - drug use and impairment of judgement - abstaining from drug needle use - clean needle use for injecting drugs - method of sterilizing unclean needles.	Participatory. Four situations involving drug or needle use are presented. Students are asked to give advice from the doctor's kit and provide reasons for that advice.
19. Are you a responsible person?	As a summary to this unit, students are asked a number of behaviour and behavioural intent questions. Behavioural intent indications may be good indicators of behaviour.	Participatory. Twelve behaviour and behavioural intent questions are asked and students respond with "yes", "no" and "not sure". A score is provided at the end to determine their personal degree of responsibility.

UNIT 2—RESPONSIBLE BEHAVIOUR—DELAYING SEX (Abstinence)

Activity	*Rationale*	*Description*
1. Reasons to say NO	It is important to stress that there are a variety of reasons for delaying sex.	Iniormational (illustrated). 10 reasons for delaying sex are given. Students participate by providing the four most common reasons for young peop]e to delay sex.
2. To delay or not to delay	Students need an opportunity to explore reasons for not having sex, and reasons why some people choose to have sex.	Participatory. An open-ended story is presented in which students explain the reasons given for having sex. Students then choose three reasons (from 10) for the male to say "no" and three for the female to say "no".
3. "Lines" and more "lines"	Students need practice in responding to typical lines that are used to pressure individuals to have sex .	Participatory. Ten lines are given and students respond with the most appropriate response from a list of 14.
4. Guidelines: help to delay sex	Students need to know that they are not alone in delaying sex. They also need help in their decision to delay sex.	Informational (illustrated). 14 suggestions are given to help students maintain their decision to delay sex. Students are asked to indicate which ones would be easy or ditficult tor them.
5. What to do?	Students need practice in using "the guidelines" for delaying sex with real-life examples.	Participatory. Three case studies are provided and students are asked to give advice that would help each person to delay sex.

6. Affection without sex?	It is unreasonable to expect young people not to show atfection during this stage of their lives. It is important to provide suggestions for alternative ways of showing affection for those who wish to delay sex.	Informational/participatory. Two hearts provide spaces tor young people to explore additional ways some are provided for them) to be affectionate without having sex.
7. What's next?	Physical affection can be very sexually arousing. The more sexually arousing the activity is, the more likely it will eventually lead to sex. Establishing limits and knowing when to express these limits is very important for young people.	Participatory. Students are asked to rank sevel physical behaviours from least to most physical. Questions are asked about limits - who; where; when.
8. Am I assertive?	Definitions of assertive, passive and aggressive behaviours are necessary to understand the verbal and non-verbal aspects of being an assertive person.	Informational (illustrated). Three people displafl the verbal and non-verbal characteristics of being assertive, passive and aggressive.
9. Who's assertive'	Recognizing assertive, passive and aggressive be haviours in real-life is necessary for a person who wants to be assertive.	Participatory. Two stories provide opportunities for students to identify the different types of behaviour.
10. Assertive messages	Students must learn specific steps to being assertive and practise those through behavioural rehearsal with actual situations involving HIV/AIDS/ STD.	Informational (illustrated). A four–step approach to being assertive is demonstrated by means of short case study.
11. Your assertive message (class)	An example of an assertive message developed by the whole class, makes it easier	Participatory. Another case study is used to encourage the class to suggest an assertive

	for individual students to develop their own message.	message using the four-step approach.
12. Your assertive message (individual)	Students must be provided with an opportunity to develop their own message.	Participatory. A choice of three case studies is provided for each student to develop a personal assertive message, using the four-step approach.
13.Responding to persuasion (demonstration)	It is extremely important that students learn to deal with people who try to distract or pressure them by persuasion to do something they think they should not do.	Informational. Ideas are given, first to deal with those who distract you from an assertive message and second, to handle those who pressure a person to do something they do not want to do.
14.Responding to persuasion (class activity)	An example of returning to your message following a distraction and dealing with persuasion makes it easier tor students to learn to deal with these problems when they develop their own strategies.	Participatory. Students learn, as a class, to return to their message if distracted. They also learn to delay, bargain or refuse if another person tries to get them to do something they do not want to do.
15. Responding to persuasion (individual)	Students learn how to deal with distracting state ments and how to be assertive when someone is pressuring them to do something they do not want to do.	Participatory. Students provide their own meassage for distracting and persuasive statements made by another person.
16: You decide	Young men and boys often have different ideas about delaying sex from young women and girls. Most of these ideas need to be	Participatory. Students are asked to respond with true or false to a number of statements dealing with gender differences. They are then

	explored and some of them need to be changed.	asked whether these differences are right or wrong. Finally, they art asked to restate the differences in a positive way.
17. Dealing with threats and violence	Women need to be aware of situations that may lead to violent sex and of individuals who may put them in such situations. They also need to leam ways of avoiding or dealing with pressures and threats to have sex.	Participatory. A case study with questions allows students to explore the many problems that may arise, and some possible solutions, when a person insists on maintaining abstinence in the face of violence and threats.
18. Being assertive every day	Students need to practise assertive skills that have been developed in the classroom in everyday life.	Participatory. Students are asked to develop a plan for being assertive outside the classroom. The plan (life management skills) involves setting goals, time lines, benefits and rewards and contract signing. They are asked to make notes on their thoughts and feelings about the activity.

UNIT 3—RESPONSIBLE BEHAVIOUR—Protected Sex

Activity	*Rationale*	*Description*
1. **The condom**	Information about condoms is necessary for effective use.	Informational: (illustrated) Provides essential information about condoms and condom use.
2. **Arguments people use against using condoms**	Although one partner may have developed positive attitudes toward condom use, they may have to deal with a partner who has negative attitudes towards condoms.	Participatory: Three responses are offered to each of 10 negative arguments about condom use. Students must select the best response for each argument.
3. **How to use a condom (explanation/ demonstration)**	One of the most important factors in condom failure is inexperience with its proper use. Therefore, an understanding of effective use of a condom is essential .	Informational (illustrated): A humorous but informational illustration of the proper steps in condom use is presented to the students.
4. **Condom practice**	The use of a model penis or other types of models to practise using a condom properly is an important activity for young people. Those who feel confident about using a condom, without appearing foolish are more likely to buy and use a condom.	Participatory (in small groups): A model penis and enough condoms for each student in the group are distributed. Using a"task card", students who wish to, follow the steps for proper condom use on the model.
5. **No to unprotected sex (demonstration)**	Using the skills learned in Unit 2 on assertive behaviour, students need to practise assertive messages to a partner who does not want to use a condom or doesn't have one to use.	Informational (illustrated): Students are shown the assertive steps of delay, bargain and refuse when a partner refuses to use a condom or persuades someone to have sex without one.

6. No to unprotected sex (class participation)	Same as Activity 5	Participation (class): the whole class participates in delay, bargain and refusal messages tor a situation where a partner is embarrassed to use a condom.
7. No to unprotected sex (individual participation)	Same as Activity 5	Participation (individual): Each person develops an assertive message with delay, bargain and refusal messages for a situation where a partner does not have a condom but wants to have sex.

UNIT 4 - CARE AND SUPPORT

Activity	*Rationale*	*Description*
1. Who discriminates?	People who are HIV positive or are living with AIDS are in many cases subject to discrimination. Young people need to be aware of discrimination and how it is expressed.	Informational/Participatory. A definition of discrimination is provided and students must provide answers to unfinished statements about discriminatory actions toward people with AIDS.
2. The story of two communities	It is important to feel what it is like to be discriminated against. This can be accomplished partially by reflecting on comments made by a person living with AIDS.	Participatory. Presents the experience of a young person living with AIDS in a very prejudiced and discriminatory community, and in a very tolerant and helpful community. Students are asked to select comments that are most hurtful and those that are most helpful.
3. Why compassion?	People who have compassion towards themselves and others are very much needed in this society. Recognizing the value of compassion is an important beginning.	Participatory. Student are asked to add to three reasons for compassion. They are then asked to discuss questions on compassion.
4. What could you do?	Students need to know ways to be compassionate and when and how to intervene.	Participatory. Students are asked to choose from a list of ways to show compassion, those that they could use to show compassion to two people—a mother with AIDS and Dwari—a schoolmate.

5. How to's of car giving	Students may have a person with AIDS in the family or neighbourhood. It is important that they know the basic norms of hygiene and home care, and that they learn ways of helping the person to cope.	Informational (illustrated). Two concepts are developed on how to provide emotional and physical care for a person with AIDS.
6. How to keep yourself safe	If you are providing care for a person with AIDS, you need to know how to care for and protect yourself.	Informational. A number of ways to protect yourself, medically and emotionally, are demonstrated in this activity.
7. What do you know?	It is useful to review information that is received passively for recall and understanding.	Participatory. A matching and a true-false test provide students with an opportunity to review information from activity 5.
8. Support for responsible behaviour	It is important to encourage young people to support peers who value abstinence or those who have made the decision to use safer sex practices (i.e. condoms) or who have shown tolerance and compassion to a person living with AIDS.	Participatory. A number of scenarios provide opportunities to support those people who have made the decision to adopt responsible, tolerant and caring behaviours.
9. Compassion, tolerance, and support	Compassion, tolerance and support mean little to young people unless they are given the opportunity to practise these behaviours in everyday situations.	Participatory. Students select from a list they have made, a situation where they can show compassion, tolerance or support. They write an action plan and journal on what happened and how they felt about the experience.

The following are the main steps in developing a curriculum for HIV/AIDS/STD education:

1. Making a situation assessment
2. Defining the type of programme
3. Selecting objectives
4. Making a curriculum plan
5. Planning for material production
6. Developing students' activities
7. Developing the teachers' guide
8. Validating the curriculum
9. Planning for teacher training
10. Designing the programme's evaluation.

Participation of parents and families in a HIV/AIDS/STD school programme, and in volving peer leaders, are issues to be considered in the design of a curriculum.

MAKING A SITUATION ASSESSMENT

In order to make a wise selection of objectives and classroom activities, it is important to gather information about your target audiences those for whom the programme is intended, and those who influence the programme or whose informed involvement is necessary. The information gathered will enable planners to develop learning materials that are relevant to the students and acceptable to most sections of the community. It will provide powerful support to advocacy about the need for AIDS education at meetings with parents and community leaders.

Students

Information that is needed about young people includes:

- Age at first intercourse, age at marriage, for boys and girls
- Age at which most leave school
- Prevalence of STD and early pregnancy
- Sources of information about sexuality
- Common beliefs about STD, contraception, marriage
- Scenarios/situations that may lead to sexual intercourse, e.g. accepting lifts from school, going to visit family members in town, boy/girlfriends proposing sex after a party or on the way to/from the market/ school, older family friends visiting, etc.
- Young people's relationships: girls' and boys' expectations, attitudes to sex, gifts for sex; forced sex; male domination

- Patterns of relationships: amongst same age; older man-young woman; young man older woman, "sugar daddies", multiple partners
- Type of sexual practices: masturbation, petting, kissing, vaginal penetration, oral sex, anal intercourse among boys and among boys and girls
- Knowledge of HIV/AIDS/STD
- Knowledge and attitudes towards condoms
- Prevalence of injecting drug use
- Extent of circumcision, tattooing, and other scarification practices
- Use of traditional healers and unqualified doctors
- Attitudes to people with HIV/AIDS.

Teachers

Information that is needed about teachers includes:

- Teaching methods most commonly used
- Reading level
- Blackboard/audio-visual equipment available
- Comfort with, and experience of teaching sexuality
- Attitudes to people with HIV/AIDS
- Familiarity with other subjects within which HIV/AIDS/STD programme could be taught
- Methods of evaluating students
- Average class size
- Attitudes to parent involvement
- Knowledge of HIV/AIDS/STD
- Willingness to teach about HIV, AIDS and STD.

Parents

Information that is needed about parents includes:

- Reading level
- Ability to understand information
- Participation in school activities
- Experience in other parent programmes
- Attitudes to people with HIV/AIDS
- Attitudes to delaying sex and providing information to young people on condoms
- Knowledge about HIV/AIDS/STD
- Acceptance of parent involvement.

Ministry of Education

Information that is needed about the Ministry of Education includes:

- Policies on HIV/AIDS/STD education
- Allotment of time for HIV/AIDS/STD programme
- Type of programme preferred: curricular or extracurricular, over one year or spread over several years
- Preferred subjects where programme can be integrated
- Method of validating new curriculum
- Willingness to evaluate the curriculum
- Expertise available in sex education, population education, family life education
- Attitudes to teacher training and time off for teacher training
- Financial resources: availability and/or constraints
- HIV/AIDS/STD education already in place.

Community

Information that is needed about the community includes:

- Prevalence of HIV/AIDS/STD, teenage pregnancy
- Availability and acceptance of condoms
- Attitudes to delaying sex
- Availability of local health and social services for people with HIV/AIDS/STD
- Ministry of Health's policies on prevention and control of HIV/AIDS
- Availability of HIV/STD testing and counselling
- Attitudes to people with HIV/AIDS
- Primary methods of transmission of HIV
- Acceptance of sexual behaviour in young people
- Attitudes and laws about injecting drug use.

How to gather information for the assessment

The following are useful sources of information forthe initial assessment:

- National AIDS Programme
- Earlier studies and reports. Check NGOs and university departments
- Individual interviews with members of key target audiences and community workers
- Rapid assessment by means of a small survey
- Focus groups. These discussions take place with 6-12 people who represent the target audience (e.g. students). A prepared list of topics is used, but facilitators encourage

participants to speak freely. The record of the discussions (notes or tape recording) provides information about the group.

- Interviews with key people in the community, such as: youth leaders, youth counsellors, community health doctors, religious leaders, public health nurses, parent/ teacher association representatives, social scientists.

DEFINING THE TYPE OF PROGRAMME

Context of HIV/AIDS/STD education

The first decision that needs to be made is where to integrate the programme.' The programme could be taught: as a separate subject or topic, as part of an established subject (e.g. population education, family life education, health education, social studies), as an extra-curricular activity, or "infused" in different subjects.

If an infusion strategy is used, maths teachers may present the statistical trends of HIV and AIDS, teachers of social studies will address the social dimensions of AIDS in the community, teachers of biology will present the biomedical aspects of HIV, AIDS, STD, teachers of religious studies will debate family values, health education teachers will address prevention, and art/ drama teachers will propose AIDS as a theme for the production of plays or posters. Materials for teachers of different subjects, and students, will have to be developed.

Having a common element running through different subjects creates an opportunity for communication and coordination among school staff; however, an infusion strategy is only recommended for mature school systems with well-trained teachers, and an efficient monitoring system that ensures implementation of the programme.

In general, science or biology are not the best carrier subjects, as they tend to place too much emphasis on biomedical aspects of HIV/AIDS/STD, at the expense of preventive, behavioural aspects.

The question of where to integrate HIV/ AIDS/STD education may require policy decisions at the higher levels of the Ministry of Education. It may be a difficult decision but it must be made early in the development of your curriculum.

Type and length of programme

The programme can be offered during one school year or divided over two to three years or more (sequential curriculum). A sequential programme is preferable, because learning can be reinforced at regular intervals; it is not as time-consuming as a one-year programme; and students are able to relate knowledge and skills to specific situations encountered at different ages.

Programmes on sexuality and HIV/AIDS/ STD education are more effective if given before the onset of sexual activity. For some countries, this may mean starting the programme in early grades. Information on age at first intercourse will greatly help planners in defining the age at which HIV/ AIDS/STD preventive education should start.

The belief that sex and AIDS education may encourage sexual activity in young people is a powerful barrier to the introduction of prevention programmes for adolescents. Yet, evidence from evaluation studies that compared groups of young people who received such education with others who did not, shows that sex and AIDS education do not promote earlier or increased sexual activity; on the contrary, sex education may lead to a delay in the onset of sexual activity, and to the use of safer sex practices among those students who are sexually active. Studies have also shown that education programmes that promoted both postponement of sexual activity and protected sex when sexually active, were more effective than those promoting abstinence alone.

Young people today are increasingly exposed to sexually explicit messages, and some are victims of sexual abuse. Parents should be the first educators, because they can grade the information according to the age and development of their children, and link it to the values they want to instil. Unfortunately, few parents talk to their children about sexual health and development. The HIV/AIDS epidemic has forced many school systems to reconsider the issue of sex education in schools, given that a large proportion of infections occur during adolescence, and that AIDS is a fatal disease.

School-leaving age is also an important factor to consider. Certainly, by the time most students leave school, they should all have received the minimum HIV/AIDS/ STD programme (see core objectives in the next section). In countries where girls tend to leave school at a younger age than boys, every effort should be made to provide AIDS-related education while they are still at school, as this might be their only chance to learn vital information for their protection.

Time allotment

Here are four aspects to be considered in making decisions about the amount of time for the programme:

- Participatory teaching methods (e.g. role playing) require more time than teacher directed methods;
- Teacher abilities and experience in AIDS or sex education;
- The amount of time the Ministry of Education and schools are willing to give to teaching the programme;
- The extent to which some topics are taught in other subjects or in the carrier subject.

The following tables show examples of programmes, ranging from 8 to 20 hours in one year to 40 hours over 3 years. Numbers indicate hours or teaching periods.

4 Examples of 1-year programmes

Programme	*prog. A*	*prog. B*	*prog.C*	*prog. D*
Unit 1 Basic knowledge	2	3	4	5
Unit 2 Responsible behaviour: delaying sex	3	3	4	4
Unit 3 Responsible behaviour: protected sex	1	2	4	6
Unit 4 Care and support	2	2	4	5
Total number of hours of instruction	8	10	16	20

2 Example of 2-year programmes

Programme	*first year*	*second year*	*total for each unit*
Unit 1	3	1	4
Unit 2	3	2	5
Unit 3	1	2	3
Unit 4	1	3	4
Total number of hours of instruction	8	8	16

Programme	*first year*	*second year*	*total for each unit*
Unit 1	4	2	6
Unit 2	3	4	7
Unit 3	1	4	5
Unit 4	2	2	4
Tatal number of hours of instruction	10	12	22

Example of a 3-year programme

Programme	*first year*	*second year*	*third year*	*total for each unit*
Unit 1	4	2	2	8
Unit 2	3	7	4	14
Unit 3	1	2	6	9
Unit 4	2	3	4	9
Total number of hours of instruction	10	14	16	40

SELECTING OBJECTIVES

Learning objectives need to be defined to guide the selection of the topics to include in the curriculum.

Objectives should be identified bearing in mind the following:

- The behaviours that put young people at risk of infection with HIV/STD that are most prevalent in your country;
- The amount of time available;
- Unit percentages of time (25%; 50%; 25%) recommended;
- Whether some topics have been taught in other subjects (e.g. Family Life Education may have a unit on delaying sex);
- Ability of students and teachers.

Examine the objectives listed below and decide whether they are realistic and adequate. In particular, consider the 11 core objectives that are proposed as a minimum requirement. Other objectives are optional. They should only be considered once the core objectives are completed. Note the student activities that cover each objective.

You will have to review the conclusions of your situation assessment study: for example, if injecting drug use is common, students will have to learn how to respond to pressures to use drugs and the importance for drug users of cleaning injecting equipment.

Core objectives

At the end of the programme, students will be able to:

Objectives	*Student activity numbers*
1. Differentiate between HIV, AIDS, STD	1.1, I .2, 1.3
2. Identify ways of transmission of HIV	1.4, 1.6, 1.7
3. Identify ways in which HIV/STD are not transmitted	1.5, 1.8, 1.9
4. Rank methods of HIV/STD prevention for effectiveness	1.10, 1.11, 1.12
5. Identify sources of help in the community	1.17
6. Discuss reasons for delaying sexual intercourse	2.1, 2.2, 2.3, 2.4, 2.5
7. Respond assertively to pressures for sexual intercourse	2.8, 2.9, 2.10, 2. 11, 2.12, 2.13, 2.14, 2.15
8. Discuss reasons and methods for having protected sex if/when sexually active	3.1, 3.2, 3.3, 3.4
9. Respond assertively to pressures for unprotected sex	3.5, 3.6, 3.7
10. Identify ways of showing compassion and solidarity towards people with HIV/AIDS	4.1, 4.2, 4.3, 4.4, 4.5
11. Care for people with AIDS in the family and community	4.5, 4.6, 4.7

Optional objectives

Objectives	Student activity numbers
12. Recognize and avoid situations that may lead to sexual abuse (accepting gifts, walking the streets, accepting car lifts, frequenting certain bars, etc.)	2.17
13. Know ways of avoiding injecting drug use and ways of preventing HIV transmission if injection drugs are used (for communities where this is a problem and there is no health education on the topic)	1.18
14. Know the progression of HIV to AIDS (signs and symptoms)	1.13, 1.14
15. Know about the procedure and counselling for testing for HIV	1.15, 1.16
16. Know alternative ways of being affectionate without having sexual intercourse	2.6, 2.7
17. Be aware of gender differences in sexual expectations	2.16
18. Be able to be assertive in everyday life situations	1.19, 2.18
19. Be able to support peers who behave in a responsible way	4.8

(No students' activities for the following objectives are included in the package)

Objectives

20. Respond assertively to pressures for sharing injecting drugs
21. Provide arguments for convincing family and friends not to go to unqualified doctors, but to use only health centres and hospitals for treatment
22. Identify the clinics and shops where condoms may be obtained or purchased
23. Seek appropriate treatment for STD
24. Discuss reasons for and against early marriage
25. Respond assertively to pressures for drinking at parties
26. Provide arguments to counteract the widespread conviction that mosquitoes spread HIV
27. Provide arguments to counteract the belief that traditional herbs can cure AIDS.

MAKING A CURRICULUM PLAN

Now that you have selected objectives that are relevant to your country, it is important to make a curriculum plan.

The following points may help you with that task:

- Objectives can be repeated at other grades if you use a sequential programme, but student activities may be different.
- Unit I - Basic Knowledge of HIV/AIDS/ STD - should be taught mainly in the early grades and emphasis on this should gradually decrease in later years, when a recap will be enough.
- Remember the time distribution: Unit I = 25%; Unit 2+3 = 50%; Unit 4 = 25% over the whole programme.
- Assess degree of difficulty of each activity - some are easier than others.
- On average, each activity takes 3/4 to I hour (depending on the ability of teachers and students).
- Generally, there will be greater acceptance of a unit on condoms, if there is a strong unit on delaying sex.
- The curriculum should include some information on condoms. Classroom activities on condoms and on saying no to unprotected sex are also strongly recommended. A graduated programme is often effective (if you use a sequential approach) - start slowly in the early grades and increase awareness in the later grades. The section on condoms will be useful in the future to those young people who are not yet sexually active, and will be useful immediately to those who already are.
- The degree of involvement of young people in Unit 4 will depend on the HIV/AIDS situation in your country. Where there are a large number of HIV/AIDS cases, and young people or their parents are expected to care for these people, an extensive unit would be advised. Take into consideration the projections for the next 5 years, and not only the present situation.
- Review the conclusions of your initial assessment study, and make sure that the activities reflect the most common situations of risk for young people in your country, both in rural and urban areas. For example, boys may be pressured by peers to have sexual intercourse to prove their maturity, or girls to prove their attachment or because they are not in a position to refuse. Activities on how to respond to these pressures will have to be part of unit 2.

A sample curriculum is illustrated below. It is a sequential curriculum for grades 6, 7, 8.

Grade level	*Objectives*	*Activities*
6	*Unit 1 (4 hours) Basic information on HIV/AIDS/STD*	
	1. Differentiate between HIV, AIDS, and STD	1.1, 1.2
	2. Identify ways of transmission of HIV	1.4, 1.6
	3. Identify ways in which HIV/STD are not transmitted	1.5
	4. Rank methods of HIV/STD prevention for effectiveness	1.10
	Unit 2 (4 hours) Responsible behaviour: delaying sex	
Approximate Age: 12 - 14	1. Discuss reasons for delaying sexual intercourse	2.1, 2.2
	2. Describe the types of assertive behaviour and the steps to a simple assertive message	2.8, 2.9, 2.10, 2.11, 2.12
	Unit 3 (I hour) Responsible behaviour: protected sex	
	1. Know basic information about condoms	3.1
	Unit 4 (I hour) Care and support for people with HIV/AIDS	
	1. Know the meaning of discrimination and how people discriminate against people with HIV/AIDS	4.1, 4.2
	Total programme time = 10 hours	
7	*Unit 1 (2 hours) Basic information on HIV/AIDS/STD*	
	1. Identify ways in which HIV/STD are not transmitted (review)	1.8
	2. Identify methods of HIV/STD prevention (review)	1.11
	3. Identify sources of help in the community	1.17
	Unit 2 (3 hours) Responsible behaviour: delaying sex	
Approximate Age: 13 - 15	1. Discuss help for delaying sex	2.5
	2. Review assertive message and learn refuse, delay, and bargain assertive messages	2.13, 2.14, 2.15
	Unit 3 (1 hour) Responsible behaviour: protected sex	
	1. Respond to arguments against condom use	3.2

	Unit 4 (2 hours) Care and support for people with HIV/AIDS	*13 - 15*
	1. Identify why it is important to be compassionate and ways of being compassionate	4.3, 4.4
	Total programme time = 8 hours	
8	*Unit 1(2 hours) Basic information on HIV/AIDS/STD*	
	1. Identify ways in which HIV/STD are not transmitted (review)	1.9
	2. Rank methods of HIV/STD prevention for effectiveness	1.12
	3. Know the progression of HIV/AIDS (signs and symptoms)	1.13
	Unit 2 (2 hours) Responsible behaviour: delaying sex	
	1 . Alternative ways of being affectionate without having sexual intercourse	2.6
	2. Recognize and avoid situations that lead to sexual abus	
Approximate Age: 14 - 16	*Unit 3 (2 hours) Responsible behaviour: protected sex*	
	1. Know the steps in using a condom correctly	3.3, 3.4
	2. Respond to pressures for unprotected sex	3.5, 3.6
	Unit 4 (2 hours) Care and support for people with HIV/AIDS	
	1. Care for people with AIDS in the family and community	4.5, 4.6, 4.7
	Total programme time = 8 hours	

Total time for sequential curriculum = 26 hours

Time by unit: Unit 1 = 8 hours (30%)
Units 2+3 = 13 hours (50%)
Unit 4 = 5 hours (20%)

PLANNING FOR MATERIAL PRODUCTION

The learning objectives and the teaching methods used in the programme will influence the type of materials needed. The programme presented in this package is largely based on participatory methods, as these are known to facilitate the learning process. The type of materials will depend on finances, and on the availability of duplicating equipment. Costs will have to be calculated carefully it is important that in countries where information materials are scarce in the community, print materials are given to students to take home, so that they can be shared with peers and family

The following alternatives may help you in your decision-making:

Materials for students

- One set of Students' Activities for each student, to be taken home to share with parents/siblings
- A set of Students' Activities (one for each student in a class) to be kept at school and used by more than one class: Students will write answers on a piece of paper rather than in the booklet
- A set of Students' Activities, one for each group of students (4 to 6) to be used in small groups
- A set of Students' Activities for each teacher or school
- A booklet for each student with essential information, to take home

Materials for teachers

- A Teachers' Guide with background information and instructions on students' activities is provided for each teacher or for each school
- Flip charts (one for each student activity) are provided for each teacher or group of teachers
- A transparency of each student activity is provided for teachers where overhead projectors are available

Materials for parents/ family members

- Please see section "Participation of parents/family members"

DEVELOPING THE STUDENTS' ACTIVITIES

One of the most important tasks at this point in your curriculum development, is to develop the student activities which best suit your culture and country. Remember that core activities should be undertaken and completed before starting on optional activities.

It is at this point that the results of your initial situation assessment will be most useful. Review the conclusions, and try to integrate the views of the young people interviewed during the initial assessment in the student activities, the words they use, and the situations in which they most often find themselves.

Most, if not all, student activities you may select from this package will have to be re-written to make them culturally relevant to the day-to-day life of young people in their community, and in particular the stories or scenarios must correspond to real risk situations.

The following checklist will help you in analysing each chosen activity and in making the necessary adaptations.

Language

- Are words understandable for the reading level of the students?
- Are sentences short with only one major thought?
- Are words used that young people are not familiar with? (it is better to use popular expressions rather than medical or scientific terms)
- Could the idea be expressed in simpler terms?
- Are medical terms limited to those that young people need to know?

Scenarios (stories, case studies)

- Are the most common risk scenarios represented, and are they appropriate to the risk situations young people experience in your country (e.g. drinking at parties, sugar daddies, anal sex with girls to avoid pregnancy, sex in exchange for small gifts, sex just to please the partner, sex to prove virility)?
- Will parents and Ministry officials approve of the scenarios you have selected?
- Should sex among males be a part of your scenarios (e.g. in some countries, boys are sought by homosexual tourists)?
- Can you include scenarios where condoms are discussed or used?
- Is sexual abuse (unwanted or forced sex) a situation that needs to be presented?
- Is it better to put names or just initials of story characters?

- Is there an equal number of boys and girls in your scenarios?
- Are the young people likely to identify themselves with the characters in the scenarios?
- Is there urban and rural representation in your scenarios? (if applicable)

Relevance to local needs

- Is there a need to consider circumcision, tattooing, scarification, and traditional healers in your educational activities?
- What sources of help for people with HIV/AIDS/STD are available? Do they include testing and counselling? Should this information be represented in the student activities?
- What are the lines/words/body language that best express assertive, passive and aggressive behaviours in the cultural groups of your country?
- Make sure local brands of condoms and lubricants are mentioned in the appropriate activities

Adaptations to meet time allotments

- Do activities need to be adapted to meet the time allotted to a specific grade? Which parts can be deleted?
- Are there aspects that you would like to add to the activities? Can you combine activities?

Illustrations

- Do you wish to use illustrations in your activities?
- Should the people be drawn as cartoons or like real people? Which would young people, parents and Ministry officials best accept?
- Which illustrations of the package can be reproduced with no or minor modifications?
- What type of clothing should people wear? What expressions should they present?
- Is there an equal number of males and females? Are different religions and ethnic groups fairly represented?
- Should affection between two males or two females be represented in the illustrations?
- Are the young people likely to identify with the illustrations presented?
- Are there urban and rural scenes represented in the illustrations?

Drawings need to be done by a professional illustrator and pre-tested with a sample of students before the final version of materials is printed.

PARTICIPATION OF PARENTS AND FAMILY MEMBERS

The involvement of parents and other family members in programmes relating to human sexuality has a beneficial effect on both students and parents.

A school-based programme needs the support of the community and family if it is to be effective. Young people are only in school for a short period of time. If the school programme is to make a difference, it needs to receive support from the home.

Parents and families who are involved in a school programme on HIV/AIDS/STD provide valuable support and motivation for the programme objectives. They may also serve as valuable resources for information and reinforcement of healthy attitudes and behaviours.

A programme that involves parents and families in an HIV/AIDS/STD programme:

- Offsets possible resistance in the community
- Increases knowledge of parents, relatives, and other children in the family, some of whom may not attend school, about AIDS.
- Ensures greater acceptance of the programme in the community
- Acknowledges the role of parents and relatives in their child's education and in the development of his or her values
- Provides support for the teacher of the programme
- Leads to closer ties between home and school on other issues
- Facilitates communication between adults and children in the family.

Although extra effort is required to produce and ensure participation of parents and the advantages are well worth the effort in terms of achieving the programme objectives.

Although many planners fear opposition by parents, most of them are favourable to programmes for the prevention of HIV/ STD, once they realize the threat that AIDS poses to their children. The need for preventive education before children become sexually active has to be explained to them; they need reassurance that sex education does not encourage sexual experimentation in adolescents, but rather, makes them aware of the risks involved.

How to involve parents and other family members

- Parents attend a parent-teacher meeting to discuss the programme, look at the materials, and ask questions (see section B-2 for a sample agenda for a parent meeting).
- Parents attend religious or political gatherings, or other community events, where the school head/principal is present, to discuss the best way to protect their children from AIDS.
- Parents might be invited to the school for a show of projects, a short play, role-play sessions, puppets, etc.
- A parents'guide can be prepared and distributed. This would provide: basic information about HIV/AIDS and about the extent of the problem in their country, particularly amongst young people; an outline of the curriculum that has been designed; and advice on how they can best help their children to learn responsible behaviours and ways to protect themselves.
- Parents are informed in writing or in a meeting, about the programme. (See section B-3 for a sample letter.)
- A leaflet is sent home to the parents explaining the programme and how they can become involved in their child's education (see section B-4 for an example).
- Students take home their completed student activity booklets to share certain activities with parents and other family members. The booklet would include an introduction to the programme and instructions to the parents (see section B-5 for an example).
- Children can ask parents questions about dating and other experiences that happened when they were young (see section B-6 for an example of these questions).

If parents are to be involved in the education programme, planners have to decide which method(s) are most suitable, and consider their cost.

One of the issues which is frequently raised in meetings with young people is their need for opportunities to discuss problems with concerned adults, since they cannot or do not want to discuss with parents or family members. Schools may organize training sessions in counselling techniques for volunteer parents, teachers and other interested community members, drawing on the expertise of health professionals, religious organizations, NGOs, and social workers. Training should cover HIV/AIDS/STD, pregnancy, sexual abuse, drug use. After training, the volunteers are available for 23 hours per week, on a roster basis. Students can visit these counsellors with the complete assurance of confidentiality.

INVOLVEMENT OF PEER LEADERS

A peer leader is a student who is selected for his/her leadership potential in helping in the education process. He/she is trained to help other students learn through demonstrations, listening, role playing, encouraging, giving feedback and supporting healthy decisions and behaviours. Note that in the Teachers' Guide, ways to use peer leaders are explained only for some activities. However, cu liculum planners and teachers should bear in mind that peer leaders may be used for almost any of the activities - whenever the teacher feels this would be useful and appropriate.

Many successful programmes have involved peer leaders. Studies have shown that:

- Young people are likely to imitate or model well-liked or respected peers
- Young people are more likely to listen to what respected peers say
- Peer leaders who exhibit healthy, responsible behaviours can influence in a positive way the behaviour of other peers
- Peer leaders can support, encourage and help their peers both inside and outside the classroom
- They can help the teacher in the classroom
- They can help manage and solve problems when students are working in small groups, particularly when the class size is large.

PEER LEADER TRAINING

Peer leaders need to be trained and supported in the many roles and responsibilities they will be expected to fulfill in the programme on HIV/AIDS/STD. Although it may take four or five hours to complete this training, the rewards in terms of programme success for teachers and students are well worth the effort.

Training will ensure that the peer leader will:

1. Understand the purpose of the HIV/ AIDS/STD programme and the importance of the peer leader's role within it
2. Be skilled in helping the teacher and students with the more difficult activities
3. Be able to help small groups of students operate effectively

4. Be a good listener, provide feedback, and be able to understand the feelings of their peers
5. Know the sources of information and counselling so that students can be referred to appropriate help.

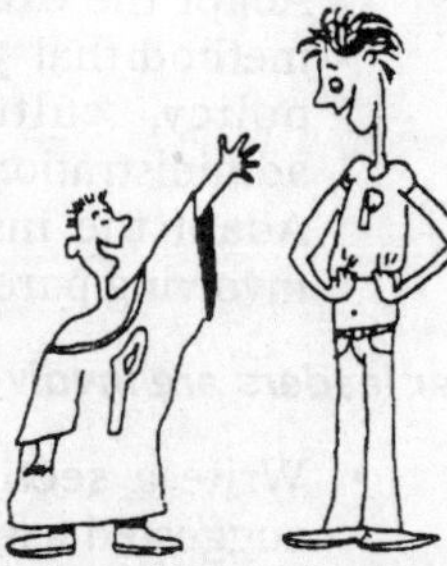

If you decide to involve peer leaders, you may consider giving them some reward for their effort, such as a cereward for their effort, such as a certificate, a partial school credit, recognition at a school or community gathering, or a T-shirt.

Peer leaders may be selected by their peers, or by the teacher, but they should not be forced into the role. They must be well-liked by other students - not seen by the classmates as the teacher's "pet". They might also be older students, who are considered opinion-leaders, are self-confident and able to listen to others. A mix of boys and girls is desirable.

DEVELOPING THE TEACHERS' GUIDE

The Teachers' Guide should be composed of the background information for teachers, and teacher instructions for each student activity selected for your curriculum.

If you take the example provided in the package as a guide, it should be modified under the following criteria:

- Language difficulty
- Type of teachers expected to use the programme
- Teaching methods decided on the basis of facilities available (blackboard, duplicating), teacher training in participatory methods, and desire to increase teacher's variety of teaching methods
- Type of materials that will be provided to students
- Sensitive issues within a country of which teachers should be aware
- Additions that would help teachers administer the programme; for example, those that result from questions that teachers asked during the initial assessment, not included in the chapter "Possible questions about HIV/AIDS/STD".

If parents and families are involved in the programme:

- Write a section on "Participation of parents and families in HIV/AIDS/STD education", with clear instructions on how to ensure participation of parents.

- Adapt the example(s) in sections B-2 to B-6, for each method that you decide to use. Reading level, school policy, cultural appropriateness, and ease of administration should be considered in your adaptation.
- Adapt the instructions to teachers for each activity involving parents.

If peer leaders are involved in the programme:

- Write a section on "Peer leaders", according to the suggested use of peer leaders
- Adapt the student activities: select those activities where peer leaders are involved, and make sure that the instructions are clear, for both the peer leaders and the teachers.

Test items for the evaluation of students

There are a number of reasons to evaluate students during and/or at the conclusion of the programme:

- To motivate students during the learning process
- To produce a grade or mark for each student
- To inform students on their progress
- To provide students with an opportunity to apply information to life situations
- To monitor learning and adjust the programme.

Section B-8 provides a wide range of questions and answers relative to each of the four units of the programme.

From these test items, you may choose those that correspond with the objectives and content of the programme. Changes in wording of the questions may be necessary, to make questions more relevant to local situations and the reading level of the students.

In particular, skills questions and life situation questions need to be carefully adapted, to provide scenarios that match real day-to-day situations as experienced by the students.

Make sure you select questions from each of the four types, and from all four units of the programme. Once the test items have been selected, they should be included in the teachers' guide.

VALIDATING THE CURRICULUM

Once your curriculum has been designed, it is important to pre-test and validate it. For the pre-test, try out the activities with students and teachers in some schools. Note the reactions of students, the skills needed by the teachers, the time needed to give the instructions and complete the activities, and the kind of class management that is most appropriate. Try the activities using different methods, e.g. group work and blackboard, group work and discussion. This exercise will make sure that the instructions you give to teachers in the teachers' guide are realistic, and take into account the availability of materials in the classroom. After the field test, revise the students' activities and teachers' guide.

A pilot programme in some 6 to 10 schools, that includes the testing at the end, is highly recommended. This is best done in collaboration with researchers from the education department of a university, or from the teacher training college.

Community acceptance is also necessary for the success of a new programme. Have the programme reviewed by:

- Students
- Parents
- Health professionals
- Representatives from various religious groups
- Teachers
- Education officials
- Social workers
- Ministry of Health officials
- People with HIV or AIDS
- Care givers to people with AIDS.

In addition to the list above, there may be others that you can identify. Decisions must be made on how many validators should be used. Too many can be unmanageable, and too few will reduce credibility of the programme. The usual procedure is to provide the selected individuals with copies of the curriculum to be reviewed and either:

a) collect their comments for consideratlon; or
b) meet as a committee to review recommendations.

This review process minimizes public opposition to the programme and provides advance publicity and support for the cur

PLANNING FOR TEACHER TRAINING

Teacher training is a crucial component of curricular innovation, particularly in the case of AIDS education, as the issues involved are extremely sensitive.

Teachers need to understand what is known about HIV/AIDS/STD so that they can give reliable information about them to students and communities; they also have to confront their own feelings, especially of fear of the disease, and about people with AIDS; they have to feel comfortable with the issues raised in the programme, particularly those related to human sexuality and sexual behaviour; and finally, they have to try out the classroom activities described in the programme.

It is strongly advised to assess the accuracy of teachers' knowledge, their attitudes and levels of comfort with sensitive topics, before designing a training programme. An instrument has to be developed to carry out the needs assessment, and section B-9 gives an example (Needs Analysis for the Teacher Training Programme) that, like others in this package, will have to be adapted to the country's needs.

Methods used in the training should reflect those expected to be used by teachers in the classroom. Presentations should be reduced to a minimum, and participants should be encouraged to share thoughts and feelings as much as possible.

An example of a 3-day teacher training agenda is included in section B-10. When possible, longer training is advisable, particularly in countries where the teachers do not have previous experience in discussing sexuality-related topics. The example will have to be adapted depending on:

- Results from the Teachers' Needs Analysis
- Length of the workshop
- Length and complexity of the curriculum
- Numbers of workshop leaders
- Current levels of teacher training and experience.

Section B-11 gives an example of an evaluation instrument to assess teachers' satisfaction with the training workshop.

DESIGNING THE PROGRAMME EVALUATION

Impact evaluation

By carrying out an impact evaluation study of the programme about HIV/AIDS/STD, the education system will be able to:

- Determine whether there have been measurable effects on the students' knowledge, attitudes, skills and behavioural intent as a result of the programme.
- Demonstrate to education officials, general public and teachers that effective programmes can be carried out.
- Make a case for obtaining additional staff or funds.
- Increase the support to the programme of teachers, parents and communities.

To measure the impact of the programme, the same test is administered to classes that do not receive the programme (control group) and to those that are taking the programme (experimental group), before the programme starts and after it is completed. A comparison between the experimental and control group will help evaluators decide whether learning is in fact associated with the programme or with other outside factors (media, parents, etc.). The control group must be similar to the experimental group and close to the numbers participating in the programme. Students in the control group will receive the programme at a later stage. There should be a central collection of the results of the tests and reassessment of the programme in light of the results.

The evaluation should be conducted by a trained evaluator experienced in sampling and the collection and analysis of data. A clear distinction between the programme developers and the evaluation research person or team should be considered: programme planners should only have responsibility for programme design, preparation and delivery; developing programme evaluation criteria and instruments; and making revisions in response to the evaluation process.

Evaluation instruments will have to be developed. An example of a Pre-Post Test Evaluation, to be given to the students in both the experimental and control groups before and immediately after the programme, is presented in this package. The model test and the scoring procedure are in *Programme evaluation instrument 1;* additional questions are listed in *Programme evaluation instrument* 2. Results from the pre-test will give useful indications to the teacher about the most common misconceptions or incorrect attitudes, and enable her/him to ensure that these issues are properly covered and given appropriate emphasis.

The model test consists of:

- 19 knowledge items, representing the eleven core objectives.
- 11 attitude statements, covering the following subjects: awareness of risks, peer pressure, abstinence, condoms, drugs, tolerance and support of people with AIDS.
- 3 skill questions on confidence to refuse sex, refuse sex without a condom, and condom use.
- 3 statements of behavioural intent.

Process evaluation

By carrying out a process evaluation study, the education system will be able to:

- Determine which programme components are most successful
- Assess the acceptability of the programme to teachers and incorporate their suggestions where appropriate
- Determine the level of difficulty of the materials and revise accordingly
- Assess the receptivity of students, peer leaders (if used), parents and administrators to the programme
- Determine the appropriateness of the teaching methods.

To measure whether the programme is effective in meeting its objectives, evaluators have to gather the opinion of teachers, parents, peer leaders (focus groups), students and school administrators, in the areas where the programme was conducted. Perceptions of the programme should be used to revise, modify and update the curriculum.

The following instruments are included in the package, that may be useful in developing your own instruments:

Teacher feedback form Programme evaluation instrument 3

- To have teachers' opinions on the student activities and corresponding teacher guide they have been using: this is an extremely important tool in the revision of the materials.

Teacher interview Programme evaluation instrument 4

- For an in-depth evaluation of the experience of teaching the HIV/AIDS/STD programme; it should be administered by trained interviewers as soon as possible after the completion of the programme.

Checklist for student focus group Programme evaluation instrument 5

- About ten students from each grade level are invited for a discussion and taped (if possible) as a group. The facilitator should not be one of their teachers; students should be allowed a great deal of freedom to explore a number of topics.

Parent interview (if parent materials were used) Programme evaluation instrument 6

- A random sample of approximately 25-30 parents per school are interviewed; make sure to get a representative sample of parents. The continuation or revision of a parent programme is dependent on the results of this evaluation.

Peer leader form and checklist for focus group (if used) Programme evaluation instrument 7

- Three or four peer leaders at each grade level are interviewed as a group to determine the effects of the peer leader programme.

School director's interview Programme evaluation instrument 8

- Often, the success or failure of a new curriculum can be influenced by the perceptions and support (or lack of support) of the school administrator.
- The director usually has perceptions about the total effect of the programme and, because of his/her experience, can often make excellent suggestions for revisions.

B

Sample Materials for Introducing the Curriculum and for Teacher Training

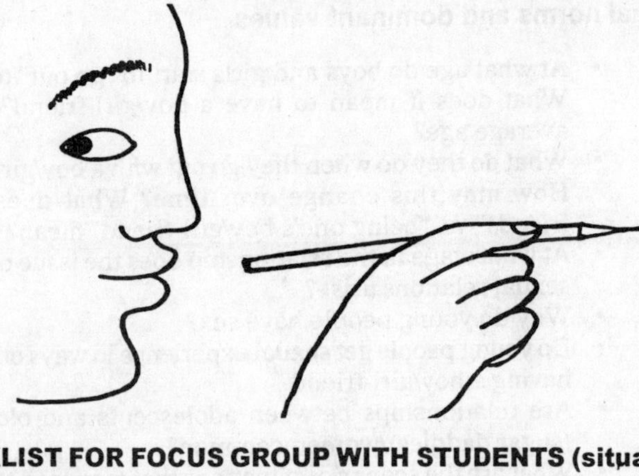

CHECKLIST FOR FOCUS GROUP WITH STUDENTS (situation assessment)

A focus group is a group discussion that gathers together people from similar backgrounds and experiences to discuss a specific topic. The participants are guided by X moderator (or facilitator) who introduces the topics in the checklist and helps the group to participate in a lively and natural discussion amongst themselves. The discussion will allow the researcher to obtain a range of understandings, views, opinions and attitudes from the group. A focus group is not an interview where participants provide individual answers. Focus groups should be conducted by facilitators trained in this method of ethnographic research.

The proceedings will be tape recorded (the preferred option), or detailed notes will be taken as the discussion progresses.

Topics for discussion with students:

Background information

- Age, sex, ethnic/language group
- With whom do they live (e.g. with family, in boarding school)?
- Do they earn any money and, if so, how?

Lifestyle and social networks

- With whom do they spend time?
- What are their leisure time activities?
- What is a typical week in their life? Is it typical of their age in their community? If not, how does it vary?
- What do they enjoy doing the most and the least?
- Do they drink? If so, how much, and in what situations?

Sexual norms and dominant values

- At what age do boys and girls start to "go out" together? What does it mean to have a boy/girl-friend? Her/his average age?
- What do they do when they go out with a boy/girl-friend? How may this change over time? What does "being friends" vs. "being one's boy/girl-friend" mean?
- At what stage in the relationship does the issue of having sexual relations arise?
- Why do young people have sex?
- Do young people get sexual experience in ways other than having a boy/girl-friend?
- Are relationships between adolescents and older men (sugar daddies)/women common?
- What are the scenarios/situations that man lead to having sex?
- What do young people mean by "havig sex" (intercourse, petting, kissing)?
- What do young people do to avoid early pregnancy (for example, anal sex)?
- Do young people experience any form of pressure to have sex? If so, from whom, Are girls forced to have sex? Do they know of cases of physical violence?
- Is having sex rewarded by gifts by the partner?
- What do people (young and older) think about having sex before marriage? What do young people think of their peers who not have sexual relations before marriage?

- How do young people learn about sex? What advice do they receive, and from whom.
- When a girl gets pregnant, what is the reaction of young people and other member of the community towards the girl and the boy? To whom can the girl turn for support?
- How is someone with many boy/girl friends considered (as successful, as model)?
- How are sexual relations among the same sex considered?
- Common beliefs about STD
- Is HIV/AIDS discussed among young people? What do people say - how are people with HIV/AIDS considered?
- Common beliefs about condoms,. contraceptives - are they easy to get?
- Are young people using drugs; inject drugs?

SAMPLE AGENDA FOR PARENT MEETING

1. Introduction of school personnel (teachers, director)

2. The need for a school programme on HIV/AIDS and STD

Examples of arguments to use for point 2:

- AIDS is a problem in our country
- Young people are at risk of getting infected with HIV/STD
- Clinics report that many young people have STD
- Young people have sexual intercourse despite the recommendations of adults to the contrary
- We do not see many young people sick with AIDS because many years pass between infection and disease - young adults with AIDS were often infected during adolescence
- Young people need information and skills to avoid infection
- Education about sex and AIDS does not encourage young people to have sex; rather, it makes them realize the risks involved;
- Parents should talk about sex with their children, and the school programme may make this easier;
- Parents are sometimes worried that their children are too young for education on sex, HIV/AIDS and STD, but times have changed, and now a days children are exposed to this information whether parents like it or not. It is better that they have the correct information;
- Sex education for delaying sex and protecting oneself from HIV/AIDS and STD is more effective if given before young people become sexually active.

3. Description of the programme

- The units and objectives
- The activities
- The parent programme (if used)

4. Questions

5. If appropriate, try one student activity with parents

6. If appropriate, show how parents/family members can interact with their children by doing an activity together

7. Final questions and farewells

SAMPLE LETTER TO PARENTS

Dear parent/guardian,

Our school is starting a new programme on AIDS education. Your child will learn about AIDS and how to protect him or herself from getting this terrible disease, and other sexually transmitted diseases.

AIDS is a problem in our country, and young people are at risk of getting injected. They need information and skills in order to avoid getting inJected. Education about sex and AIDS does not encourage young people to have sex; rather it makes them realize the risks involved and enables them to make responsible decisions about delaying sex or protecting themselves. Studies have shown that this kind of education is most effective if given before young people become sexually active.

Your interest and support in these activities will be most valuable. If you have any questions about the programme do not hesitate to contact me.

Yours sincerely,

(Name of school director, teacher, or secretary of school board)

SAMPLE INTRODUCTION TO PARENT ACTIVITIES

Dear parent/guardian,

Your son/daughter will be part of a new programme at school about AIDS and other sexually transmitted diseases. He/she will learn important information and skills to help prevent him/her from becoming sick with these serious diseases. For example:

[add here a brief description of the programme]

It is important for you to help your son/daughter with his/her learning. You can do this by:

- *Asking your child what he/she learned at school about AIDS and other sexually transmitted diseases.*
- *Reviewing activities that have been done at school with your child (or activities that will be sent home with your child).*
- *Discussing how you feel about these serious diseases.*
- *Listening carefully and calmly when he/she wants to talk about the subject.*

Thank you for your help.

Yours sincerely,

(Name of school director, teacher, or secretary of school board)

SAMPLE INSTRUCTIONS TO PARENTS

Your son/daughter has been part of a new programme at school about HIV/AIDS and other sexually transmitted diseases. He/she has completed a number of activities which are contained in the booklet your child has brought home. We advise you to review the booklet with him/her. This will provide you with the opportunity to play a part in your child's education and the development of his/her values. Included in this letter is a list of questions that you may want to ask your son/daughter about HIV/AIDS/STD and the programme he/she is taking at school.

How to talk to your child about HIV/AIDS and STD

- Read the booklet on your own
- Select a quiet time when you and your son or daughter have time to talk
- Start with one easy activity example page
- Have your child read the information to you
- Listen carefully and calmly. Ask for and listen to your child's feelings and opinions
- Try to avoid "preaching" to your child but be sure to express your feelings and opinions
- If you or your child feel uncomfortable, stop and try again at another time.

Note: Your involvement in these activities with your son/daughter is completely voluntary. There is no penalty to your child for not doing these activities. However, if you take an interest in the programme he/she is taking at school, it will make the learning easier for your child.)

Questions to ask regarding HIV/AIDS/STD

General questions

1. What did you learn about AIDS today/ this week/during the course?
2. What was the most interesting part of the lesson/course?
3. What was the most important information that you learned?
4. What did you think about the lesson?
5. What did the other students think, say, feel, about these topics?
6. Were you able to understand the activity? What did you find easy or difficult?
7. Would you read the activity to me and explain the information?
8. Maybe we can do the activity together and you can help me with the questions and answers.
9. What do you think is important for me to know?
10. How does the information apply to you?

Specific questions:

1. What is AIDS; sexually transmitted diseases?
2. How does one get HIV or AIDS?
3. How can you avoid getting infected?
4. How is one tested for HIV?
5. How do you know if someone has AIDS?
6. What happens if you live close to someone with AIDS?
7. Is there a cure for AIDS?

Other questions:

1. How do you think a person would feel if he/she had HIV/ AIDS?
2. What things could you do to help a person with AIDS?
3. How would you feel if there was someone in your class with HIV?
4. Why are people with AIDS sometimes treated unkindly?
5. Are you frightened about the AIDS situation? If yes, why?

SAMPLE QUESTIONS STUDENT TO PARENT

We can always learn from past experiences. What your parents experienced when they were younger can be a valuable lesson for you

1. If they are willing, interview your parents, or another adult relative, with the questions listed below.

2. Interview them separately.
3. You may only want to select certain questions to ask them.
4. Write their responses on a piece of paper.

Possible questions:

1. Who in your family/community talked to you about sex when you were young?
2. How old were you?
3. What did they tell you?
4. If nobody talked to you about sex, would you have liked them to? Why?
5. Do you think it was accurate / useful information?
6. How would you have liked to have received your sex education?
7. How old were you when you had your first boy/girlfriend?
8. What did you do when you spent time with him/her?
9. Did you think about birth control when you were young? Why or why not?
10. Did girls ask boys out? Do you think this would be all right today?
11. Did boys give presents to girls? Why?
12. What STDs were a concern during your youth ?
13. How did your friends protect themselves from them?
14. If you could change things, would you do things differently? Which things?

PEER LEADER TRAINING GUIDE

This guide is written for you to follow during your training session. You have been selected to be a peer leader for a health education programme on HIV/AIDS and STD, and asked to help in a variety of class activlties. The skills you will learn during this training will help you in many future situations in your life.

Who is a peer leader?

A peer leader is a person who is selected for his/her leadership potential in helping others. A peer leader is trained to help other students learn through demonstrations, listening, role playing, encouraging, giving feedback and supporting healthy decisions and behaviours.

Why are peer leaders important?

Because:

- Young people are likely to listen to, and imitate, peers that are well-liked and respected

- Peer leaders who give examples of healthy behaviours can influence behaviours of other peers and help them to avoid taking risks
- Peer leaders can support, encourage and help their peers both inside and outside the classroom
- Peer leaders can help the teacher in presenting the lesson, allowing more time for other activities and more individual attention
- Peer leaders can help manage and solve problems when students are working in small groups.

Training programme objectives

As a result of this training programme, you, as a peer leader, will:

- Understand the purpose of the HIV/ AIDS/STD education programme, and the importance of the peer leader's role within it
- Be able to help the teacher and students with some activities
- Be able to help small groups of students work together effectively
- Be a good listener, provide feedback, and be able to understand the feelings of your peers
- Know other sources of information and counselling so that you can refer your peers to appropriate help.

Each of the next sections will provide information and activities to help you achieve the objectives of this peer leader training session.

Purpose of the HIV/AIDS/STD education programme

In this programme you will learn about STD, HIV and AIDS, examine attitudes about delaying sex and using condoms, feelings about people who have HIV/ AIDS, and reasons that young people take risks with their health and their lives. You will also learn skills: (1) how to be assertive so that you say "no" to things you do not wish to do, especially to say "no" to sex or "no" to sex without a condom; and (2) to use a condom effectively.

Activities where you can help

The following is a small selection of activities with which you can help. Read them and your teacher will explain to you how you will help in the classroom.

Unit	Activity No.	Name of activity	Explanation/ demonstration
1	1.9	Are you at risk?	
		Part 1	Demonstration
		Part 2	Explanation
		Part 3	Explanation
2	2.10-2.12	Assertive messages	Demonstration
	2.13-2.15	Responding to persuasion	Explanation
3	3.3-3.4	Condom practice	Demonstration
4	4.4	What could you do?	Explanation

Helping small groups

Basic group rules

When helping small groups, use the following group rules to encourage discussion and participation:

- No put-downs (negative comments)
- Only one person talks at a time; no interrupting of others
- Everyone has a right to "pass" (to decline to discuss a personal issue)
- Everyone is given an opportunity to talk
- Keep on the topic; no side discussions on other topics; and
- "What you hear stays here" (information is confidential).

Dealing with problem situations in groups

In small groups, not every group member may be willing to complete the activity. You should be prepared to help solve minor communication problems that might arise in small groups, e.g. when a member of the group:

- Dominates the conversation (the dominator)
- Is critical of others; puts other people down, usually to make himself/herself feel superior
- Tells others what to do all the time
- Often interrupts other people
- Does not participate in the group activity
- Chats about things not related to the activity.

Ways of dealing with problems in groups

- If there are disruptions, politely remind the group that there is a problem or task to solve as well as a time limit
- Talk privately to the person causing the problem. Review the basic group rules and how the person's behaviour is negatively affecting the group. Request his/her support and cooperation for the next time the group meets

- Respond to those who interrupt by saying, "Excuse me. Just a reminder that everyone in the group has the right to speak without being interrupted"
- If the behaviour is so disturbing that it cannot be ignored, deal with it in the group. Criticize *what is* being said or done (*not the person* responsible for the disruption or making disruptive statements). Point out how the behaviour blocks the group from functioning well
- At the end of a group session, lead a discussion of how the group is doing. Try to do this in such a way that feelings are not hurt.

Now, in a small group, complete the activity "Dealing with problems in groups".

Group exercise - Dealing with problems in groups

1. On your own, read each of the situations below:
2. Brainstorm in your group a number of solutions to each situation. If you need help, review "Helping small groups"
3. Decide as a group on the best solutions and write them in the spaces provided
4. Answer the Follow-up questions. Discuss answers in your group.

Situation	*Solution*
Situation 1 The small group has been together for a few days now and it is quite clear that Dominico dominates the others. He talks most of the time and when others say something, he does not pay attention.	
Situation 2 Laura had been very quiet during the first group meeting. However, suddenly she becomes very critical of the other group members. She made rude remarks to one person in particular but also objected to opinions expressed by the rest of the group.	
Situation 3 Jaloni is a little older than the others in the group because he failed an earlier grade. He tells people in his group what to do and how to do it. No one has objected to what he is doing but you can tell they are not happy about the situation.	
Situation 4 Helena often interrupts others in the group. She	

also puts others down by calling their ideas "stupid", or "dumb". The rest of the group is getting angry with her because of her behaviour in the group.	
Situation 5 Bonois is not really interested in the class. When he is in his group he acts "bored" and seldom makes any suggestions to the group. At other times he tries to talk to someone in the group about something completely off topic. If others do not join him he becomes loud and disruptive.	

Follow-up questions

1. Which 2 of the 5 situations would be most difficult to deal with? Why?
2. Do you think you could deal with these 2 situations? Why or why not? If not, what would you work on to deal with them better?
3. Discuss ways of reinforcing or supporting someone who is trying to change problem behaviour in a group working on a task.

Communication skills

Since you will be working with other students, it is important that you ensure that you have good communication skills. You probably already have many of these skills to some extent because you have been selected as a peer leader; however, three skills which most people need to continue to improve are listening actively, giving feedback, and showing empathy (showing you understand how the other person feels or what his/her point of view is).

Listening well

To listen well so that you really hear and understand what another person is saying means that you:

- Focus on the person with direct eye contact (looking into people's eyes)
- Do not interrupt
- Do not cut in to descnbe your experience
- Do not give your attention to outside disruptions (other people or events)
- Are comfortable with silence.

After reviewing these points, complete the activity "Communication check".

Communication check

1. Rate each of the following skills using the key below:
1 = Never; 2 = Sometimes; 3 = Often; 4 = Always

1. I do not interrupt others in my group
2. My voice is appropriately pitched (not squeaky, loud or too soft)
3. I do not dominate the conversation (giving others a chance to speak)
4. I talk an equal amount compared to others
5. I look people in the face
6. I do not criticize (put down) others
7. When listening, I show my reaction to the speaker (e.g. by nodding)
8. I express what I feel, not only what I think
9. I face the speaker and avoid crossing my arms or turning away from him/her
10. I ask (encourage) others to speak
11. I respond to the speaker, showing interest
12. I do not interrupt others to make my point
13. I pay attention to the speaker the whole time he/she is talking
14. I ask questions to show interest in what the speaker is saying.
15. I criticize what a speaker says and how he/she says it rather than judging the speaker himself/herself

Total score

2. Add your scores for the items and identify where you stand on the summary score below:

Communication skills: summary score

15-27 points = Poor; 28-39 points = Fair; 40-47 points = Good; 48-60 points = Excellent

3. List your communication strengths:

4. List the communication skills you need to work on:

Follow-up questions

1. Share some of your communication strengths and weaknesses with a group member
2. Discuss what each of you could do to help work on the weaker communication skills.

Giving feedback

To give feedback to another person means you comment on the person's statements behaviour or performance. When you do this, you show the other person that you are listening and care about what he/she has said or done.

Do

- Ask questions to show you are interested in the person (e.g. "How do you feel about that?")
- Be sincere, caring and understanding
- Use verbal encouragement (such as "What happened then?")
- Use nonverbal encouragement (such as nodding your head)
- Ask questions to make the situation clearer (if necessary)
- Summarize the person's points and feelings

Do not

- Judge the person
- Comment on things that cannot be changed
- Interrupt too early to give feedback

Sources of support

You may have the opportunity to talk privately with students who need information or counselling that you cannot give them. Therefore, it is important for you to know where you can get help in your community. With your teacher, your group of peer leaders should identify a number of sources and how to reach them. These sources will enable students to get information about HIV/AIDS/STD; to obtain medical help; to go for counselling; and to be tested for HIV.

Suggestions for your list are as follows:

- Doctors
- Clergy
- Medical centre
- Health clinic
- Counsellor
- Church groups
- Places where you can get or buy condoms
- Nurses
- AIDS hotline
- Hospital
- STD clinic
- Social worker
- Youth groups
- Teacher

With your teacher, also discuss when to refer a person and specifically who the best source(s) would be for a particular situation.

TEST ITEMS FOR STUDENT EVALUATION (WITH CORRECT ANSWERS)

True-False questions

Please note that those marked with (*) are particularly recommended for inclusion in short tests.

Unit 1

		T = True F = False
1.	A person can "pass" an HIV test, that is, be negative, but still be infected with HIV.	T
2.	Men may pass HIV on to others through their semen.	T
3.	You may get HIV by sitting on a toilet seat that a person with AIDS has used.	F
4.	You may get HIV from drinking from the same glass or water fountain that a person with AIDS drank from.	F
5.	HIV is found in semen, vaginal fluids, and blood.	T
6.	A person may get HIV by sharing drug needles.	T
7.	People infected with HIV are usually very thin and sickly.	F*
8.	Once you are infected with HIV, you are infected for life.	T*
9.	Some people have been infected with HIV by swimming in the same water as someone with AIDS.	F
10.	You may get HIV from a mosquito bite.	F*
11.	Someone with AIDS can spread HIV by coughing and spitting.	F
12.	There is no way to kill HIV on a drug needle.	F
13.	Women may pass HIV on to others through their vaginal fluids.	T
14.	There is no way you can find out if you are infected with HIV.	F
15.	You may get infected with HIV by having sex with someone who shares drug needles.	T
16.	It is not dangerous to hug a person with AIDS.	T*
17.	People infected with HIV do not necessarily look sick.	T
18.	You can be cured of AIDS if you are careful to take medicine the doctor gives you.	F
19.	You can't get HIV from sharing needles for tattoos or ear/nose piercing.	F
20.	People with AIDS die from serious diseases.	T
21.	It is difficult for women to get HIV/AIDS.	F
22.	HIV may be passed from a mother to her unborn or newborn baby.	T*
23.	HIV may be spread by wearing clothes from a person with AIDS.	F*
24.	A person may get HIV by donating blood.	F*

25. Having sex during the menstrual cycle increases the risk of getting HIV. T
26. You may get HIV by cutting the skin with a knife or razor blade used by someone with HIV. T
27. The time from getting HIV until a person becomes sick with AIDS can be as short as 6 months to as long as 10 years or more. T*
28. A person who has AIDS usually will die in 6 months to 2 years. T*
29. A person is infectious (able to pass HIV on to others) only when she/he has AIDS F
30. The reason that you see so few teenagers with AIDS is that it takes years for AIDS to develop after a person has been infected. T
31. The test for HIV (ELISA test) is looking for the HIV virus. T
32. A vaccine is available to protect people from HIV infection. F
33. If a person has an STD, his or her chances of being infected with HIV are increased. T
34. AIDS is caused by HIV. T
35. There have been reported cases in which HIV was spread by kissing. F
36. A person who has tested positive for HIV is said to have AIDS. F*
37. HIV is not spread from one person to another through daily activities. T
38. There is evidence that some insects can actually spread AIDS. F
39. Teenagers infected with HIV when they are 14 may not show any AIDS symptoms until they are in their middle twenties. T
40. HIV can be spread by contact such as hugging, kissing or holding hands. F
41. A person may pass on HIV even though he/she has no signs or symptoms of AIDS. T
42. The more partners a person has, the greater the chances of being infected with HIV. T
43. Everyone infected with HIV, whether they have symptoms of AIDS or not, can spread HIV to others. T
44. A person can have HIV for years without getting AIDS. T
45. You can tell if a person has HIV by how they look. F
46. A negative HIV test means there are no antibodies to HIV in the blood. T
47. You may get HIV from toilet seats. F

48. Married people don't become infected with HIV. F
49. If you only have sex with people who look healthy, you won't become infected by HIV. F

Unit 2

T = True
F = False

1. Delaying sex and not using injecting drugs are very good ways for teenagers to avoid getting HIV. T
2. One way to avoid getting HIV is by not having sex. T
3. There is no way to protect yourself from HIV/AIDS. F
4. Not having sexual intercourse is the most effective way to avoid being infected with HIV. F
5. An example of showing affection without sex is cuddling and caressing. T
6. Assertive people get their way by overpowering others. F
7. Aggressive people get what they want without any thought about the feelings of the other person. T
8. A passive person often gives in to what others want.
9. If a person tries to get you to do something you don't want to do, you should refuse, or bargain safer alternatives, or delay the decision. T* T
10. if you stick to one partner you won't become infected with HIV. F*

Unit 3

1. You can't get HIV if you only have sex once or twice without a condom. F*
2. Condoms offer complete protection against HIV. F
3. Vaseline is a very good lubricant to use with a condom. F
4. Condoms used correctly and every time one has sexual intercourse, protect from HIV and STD and prevent pregnancy. T*
5. Lubricated condoms break more often than those that are not lubricated. F
6. If a condom slips off in the female vagina she will become sick. F
7. A condom can be safely reused. F*
8. It is important to keep condoms in a warm, moist place. F

Unit 4

1. You can get HIV by eating food prepared by an HIV infected person. F
2. A person with AIDS who has sweating, vomiting and diarrhoea needs extra fluids. T*
3. People with AIDS should stay in hospitals all the time, not at home. F*
4. People who are ill with AIDS should be encouraged to do what they can for themselves. T
5. There have been no cases of HIV from living with a person who has HIV or AIDS T
6. A person with HIV who is not allowed to attend school is an example of discrimination. T*

Short answer questions

Acceptable answers are in italics

Unit 1

1. Name three body fluids that are known to spread the AIDS virus, HIV.
   - *Male semen; vaginal secretions; blood*
2. Name two ways in which blood-to-blood transmission of the AIDS virus, HIV, can occur.
   - *Sharing injection needles and syringes; sharing other instruments - knives, razor blade. tattooing and ear-piercing instruments and possibly toothbrushes; blood transfusions*
3. What are three ways HIV is spread?
   - *Sexual intercourse; sharing injection needles and syringes and other cutting instrumen (e.g. knives); mother to baby; blood transfusion*
4. Give two reasons why AIDS is so serious.
   - *No cure for AIDS*
   - *No vaccine to prevent HIV*
   - *Causes death*
   - *Happens to young people*
   - *Discrimination and intolerance*
5. List five ways by which HIV is *not* spread.
   - *Insects, hugging or touching, towels, Spitting, coughing, sneezing, kissing; sharing a bud house, room; animals; wearing old clothes; cigarettes; swimming pools (hot tubs); telephones shaking hands; food, dishes; toilet seats; giving blood; water fountains*

6. List four ways that you can protect yourself from HIV and other infections.
   - *Not have sexual intercourse*
   - *Delay sex*
   - *Use a condom properly*
   - *Do not use dirty injection needles or syringes*
   - *Get injections only at hospitals or health centres*
   - *Have only one sexual partner who is not infected with HIV/STD and has no other sexual partners*

7. Describe what happens from the time a person is infected with HIV to the time he/she dies from AIDS.
   - *Infected with HIV; 2 to 12 weeks: antibodies develop; about 6 months to 10 years or more: symptoms start to appear, AIDS; about 6 months to 2 years or more: death*

8. What is meant by the "window period?" Why is this period so important?
   - *"Window period" is the period of time from when a person is infected until antibodies (germ fighters) develop in the blood. This is usually 2 to 12 weeks. It is important because if one is tested during this period, the test will be negative since the test looks for antibodies against HIV, which have not formed yet. However, the person can infect others.*

9. How do people look and feel from the time they are infected with HIV to the time they die from AIDS?
   - *The person may look healthy and feel fine for a long time after she/he gets infected - Then, she/he starts having swollen glands, fever, night sweats, fatigue, cough - Then serious diseases may occur- T.B., cancer, lung disease, brain illnesses, fungal infections. These result, eventually, in death.*

10. Give three reasons why a person might want to get tested.
    - *Not to infect others - Not to pass HIV on to her baby*
    - *To get treatment which may help to prevent*
    - *Not to give infected blood opportunistic infections such as pneumonia*
    - *To tell her/his sexual partners*

11. What two pieces of advice could you give to a person who injects drugs?
    - *Never share needles or syringes with anyone else*
    - *Stop using injecting drugs*
    - *Turn used needles in for clean ones*

- *Clean used needles with bleach (1 part bleach to 10 parts water)*
- *Seek help from professionals*

12. List three sources of help that a person could use if they were worried about HIV/ AIDS.
    - *Parents; doctor; teachers; counsellor; social worker; STD clinic; nurse; religious leaders; health centre; AIDS hotline*

Unit 2

13. Give four reasons for saying "no" to sex or for delaying sex.
    - *Pregnancy*
    - *You have drunk too much*
    - *Risk of STD orAIDS*
    - *Your religion says "no"*
    - *Parents don't want you to have sex*
    - *You' re not ready*
    - *Not with the right person*
    - *Want to wait until marriage*
    - *Fear of violence*
    - *Time for friendship to develop*

14. List three things that could help a person to delay sex.
    - *Go out with a group of friends*
    - *Decide early how far you want to go*
    - *Decide on your alcohol/drug limits*
    - *Don't fall for romantic words and arguments*
    - *Be very clear about your limits*
    - *When feeling uncomfortable - leave*
    - *Get involved in activities (sports, clubs)*
    - *Don' t go around with people who pressure you to have sex*
    - *Be honest from the beginning about your sexual limits*
    - *Don't go out with people you cannot trust*
    - *Avoid lonely spots where you couldn't get help*
    - *Don' t accept rides from those you can' t trust*
    - *Don't accept money and presents from people you don't know very well*
    - *Avoid going to someone's room when there is no one else at home*
    - *Express affection without having sexual intercourse*

15. Give three ways a person could be affectionate to a partner without having sexual intercourse.
    - *Hold hands* - *Say "I like (love) you"*

- *Kiss*
- *Hug*
- *Touch*
- *Massage*
- *Masturbate*
- *Write a letter*
- *Body rub*

16. How does "the mountain climbing" idea help you to make decisions about your sexual limits?
    - *The farther you go the more difficult it is to stop.*
    - *It is difficult to go back to a safer point.*
    - *Decisions about sexual limits should be made at a point where you know it will not lead to sexual intercourse.*

17. Describe the characteristics of passive, assertive and aggressive persons.
    - Passive persons
    - Do not stand up for their own rights
    - Put others first at their own expense
    - Give in to others
    - Always apologize
    - Remain silent when something bothers them

    Assertive persons
    - Respect self and other people
    - Listen and talk
    - Express positive and negative feelings
    - Are confident but not "pushy"
    - Stand up for own rights without putting others down
    - Use "I feel " statements

    Aggressive persons
    - Have no thought for other people
    - Put self first at expense of others
    - Overpower others
    - Argue
    - Get what they want at the expense of others

18. What are the advantages of being assertive?
    - Can say "no " without feeling guilty
    - Disagree without becoming angry
    - Ask for help when needed
    - Feel better about yourself
    - Avoid arguing
    - Have morefriends
    - Have better relationships
    - Have respect for yourself
    - Others will respect you

19. List three things a person could do to prevent sexual threats and violence.
    - *Be assertive*
    - *Set sexual limits early*
    - *Avoid secluded (lonely) spots*
    - *Do not accept money or presents*
    - *Do not go to person's room if no one else is at home*
    - *Do not take rides with strangers*

Unit 3

20. Give three reasons why a sexually active person would not use a condom to protect against HIV and/or pregnancy.
    - *no money or no place to get them*
    - *didn't have one at the time*
    - *use of alcohol or drugs - unable to make wise decisions*
    - *"nothing can happen to me"*
    - *takes risks to make wise decisions*
    - *embarrassed to buy or use condoms*

21. What three things would you look for in a good condom?
    - *lubricated*
    - *expiry date or date of manufacture*
    - *tip to catch semen*
    - *made of latex*
    - *package easy to open*
    - *instructions with package*
    - *diagrams on how to use a condom*
    - *spermicide added*
    - *no light goes through package*

22. What is the most important step in using a condom to prevent it from being left in the female vagina?
    - *hold rim of condom when withdrawing the penis from the vagina*
    - *remove penis from vagina before erection is lost*

23. Name two things that could be done to reduce the chance of a condom breaking.
    - *use water-based lubricant*
    - *don't use past expiry date*
    - *pinch air from tip of condom*
    - *smooth condom out after it is on*
    - *never reuse a condom*
    - *be careful when opening the package*
    - *put condom on properly*
    - *store condoms in cool, dark spot*

be careful in taking condom off

24. What could a person do if a condom did break?
    - *withdraw penis immediately*
    - *have another condom available*
    - *the woman should not douche - she should wash and urinate as soon as possible*
    - *use spermicide if possible*

Unit 4

25. Give an example of discrimination
    - *a person is not given a job because she/he comestrom another religion or culture*
    - *women aren 't paid as much as men even when they do the same job*
    - *a person with HIV is not allowed to swim with others*

26. Give two reasons why it is important to be compassionate to a person with HIV or AIDS
    - *they are often young*
    - *they will likely die*
    - *they are no threat*
    - *it is a painful, long-term disease*
    - *they suffer more if isolated*
    - *they are often abandoned by family and friends*
    - *it is important to think of someone other than yourself*

27. What are four ways to be compassionate to a person with HIV or AIDS?

- *Write a letter (note)* - *Celebrate special days*
- *Share a meal* - *Get medicines*
- *Clean the house* - *Share emotions- laugh, cry*
- *Give them a hug* - *Do not let them blame themselves*
- *Just listen* - *Be friendly*
- *Make a "fun" present* - *Play games*
- *Help other family members* - *Hold their hand*
- *Find others to give support* - *Talk about the future*

28. What could a person do to give support to a person who has AIDS and:

    a) *has loss of appetite?*
    - *Ask what they would like to eat, when and how much*
    - *Eat with the person when possible*

    b) *is vomiting?*
    - *Prepare small meals with little fat*

- *Encourage them to drink liquids*
- *Advise them to avoid food when feeling nauseated*

c) *has body sores from being in bed?*
- *Change sleeping position often*
- *Encourage short walks and sitting in chair*
- *Wash sores*

29. Give three ways you can protect yourself if you are looking after a person with AIDS.
- *Use bleach and soap and use gloves to clean soiled clothes or bedding*
- *Wash hands with warm, soapy water after contact with infected person*
- *Put used needles and syringes in hard plastic or metal box*
- *Wash thermometers with soap and water*
- *Keep cuts, sores or rashes covered at all times*
- *Clean bathroom with bleach*
- *Clean dishes with hot, soapy water*

NOTE: You should wear a mask if you are ill so as not to infect the person with AIDS.

30. Provide three ways that you can give emotional support to people with AIDS.
- *Find out about their needs and what they can do for themselves each day*
- *Share feelings - be honest and open*
- *Encourage them to do as much as possible for themselves*
- *Give support and praise when deserved*
- *Ask them how they want things done - wash, food, cleaning*
- *Encourage anger and crying*
- *Look after yourself - take breaks, ask for help*

Skill questions

The steps on the left side of the box are already filled in; the right side of the box is left blank. There are example statements in italics, but answers will vary from student to student.

1. For the situation described, write an assertive script in the empty part of the "Script box".

Situation: Your boyfriend/girlfriend becomes jealous when you are with other friends, including those of the other sex, and wants you to spend less time with them. You do not want to lose your friends and decide to tell your boyfriend/girlfriend how you feel and that you are not ready to give up your friends.

Script box:

1. Explain your feelings and the problem.	*I feel upset when I 'm pressured not to see my friends.*
2. Make a request.	*My friends are important to me and I'd like it better if you would make them your friends too.*
3. Ask how the other person	*Do you think you could do that for me?*
feels about your request.	

Response: I *guess I'm a little jealous, so I'll try to make them my friends too.*

4. Accept with thanks.	*Thanks for understanding. Let's go for a walk.*)

2. For the situation described, write an assertive refuse, delay and bargain message in the empty part of the "Script box".

Situation: You are at a party with friends. They are drinking beer and offer you one. You really don't want the beer and tell them so. They continue to pressure you to drink and finally you respond with a refusal, bargain and delay response.

Script box:

1. Explain your feelings and the problem.	*I feel angry when I say I don 't want a beer and I 'm still pressured to have one.*

They make a distracting statement: You really get red when you're angry.

2. You get back on topic	*Please let me finish what I was saying.*
3. Make a request.	*Could you please just accept that / don't want a beer tonight?*
4. Ask how the other person feels about your request.	*Is that OK with you ?*

They make a persuasive statement: Well, what are you here for if you don't want to drink?

5. You refuse	Look, I'm not going to drink and I am having a good time.
6. Delay	Look, I'll think about it, we'll see later
7. Bargain	Look, let's have a dance instead of arguing about the beer.

3. For the situation described, write an assertive refuse, delay and bargain message in the empty "Script Box" for a person who does not want to wear a condom.

Situation: You are going out with a person you really like. She/he wants to have sexual intercourse with you but does not want to use a condom. You will only have sex if a condom is used and you have a condom with you.

Script box:

1. Explain your feelings and the problem.	*I feel upset when you say you don't want to use a condom especially when I have one with me.*

He/she makes a distracting statement: Look, don't try to tell me what to do.

2. You get back on topic 3 Make a request	*Please let me finish what I was saying. I'm not trying to tell you what to do. I'm saying that I won't have sex with you without using a condom.*
4. Ask how the other person feels about your request.	*Is that all right with you?*

He/she makes a persuasive statement: They just don't feel good and it would probably break anyway.

5. You refuse	*No sex without a condom and I mean it.*
6. Delay	*Well, I guess we'll have to talk about this more.*
7. Bargain	*What could we do that would make us both happy?*

4. Arrange the following list of steps to use a condom in the correct order, by placing the number (1, 2, 3, etc.) from the column "Condom steps" beside the number in the right-hand column "Correct order of steps."

Condom steps	Correct order of steps
a) Squeeze air from tip	3 or 4
b) Unroll condom - slide it off	8
c) Open package	1
d) Roll condom on penis	5
e) Point condom the right way	2
f) Hold rim of condom and withdraw	7
g) Dispose of condom	9
h) Position the condom on the glans of the penis	3 or 4
i) Smooth out and add lubricant	6

Life situation questions

1. *Dacobi and Kandu are close friends but live in different towns. They often visit each other and on one visit, Kandu asks Dacobi how AIDS is prevented. Dacobi has had a few classes about AIDS in school but can't remember everything he was taught. However, he does tell Kandu what he knows about prevention. Some of what he says is not true. Mark an "F" for these statements. Mark "T" for those statements that are true.*

a)	It is easy to tell who has HIV and who hasn't, so you don't need to worry about using a condom to avoid infection.	F
b)	HIV is only present in certain body fluids, mainly male semen, vaginal secretions and the blood. Therefore, don't have sex without a condom and don't use needles or other sharp instruments that might have someone else's blood on them.	T
c)	Be careful of mosquitoes and other insects that bite as that is a way HIV is spread.	F
d)	The only really safe way to protect yourself is to delay sex until you are ready to take the responsibility of using a condom.	T
e)	A blood test for HIV is the only way to tell if you have been infected with HIV.	T

2. *Aaren and Mayada have decided to have sexual intercourse. Both have had sexual intercourse before without using a condom but are confident that none of their previous partners had a disease. Mark "T" for any statements that are true/correct and "F" for any statements that are not true/false.*

a)	If they have sex, it will be all right because HIV cannot be spread until a person has AIDS.	F
b)	If they have sex, Aaren should wear a condom every time they have sexual contact.	T
c)	They would know if their previous partners had HIV.	F
d)	They would be safe if they had oral or anal sex without a condom.	F
e)	They would be safer if they delayed sex until they were both properly tested.	T

3. *You are talking with three of your same-sex friends about "lines" young people use to get "sex." The group decides to try to come up with good responses to these "lines". What would you say in response to the following lines:*

Line:	Response:
"Everyone does it." "I'll buy you something nice if you let me do it." "We don't have to worry about AIDS, I haven't got it." "This is the first time I've had sex. I can't have a disease." "Either we do it, or we're through."	The teacher should use her/his judgement as to correct responses. (see Unit 2/ Student activity 3)

4. *Ranjki is a person who will be going to your school next year and everyone knows that he has HIV. He is not sick now and he is really looking forward to entering his new school. List four things you could do to show compassion and support for Ranjki when he arrives at your school.*
   - Stay with him during breaks.
   - Go to his place and welcome him to your school.
   - Walk to school or from school with him.
   - Ask him to sit near you.
   - Be in the same group when possible.
   - Get other students to help support Ranjki.

5. *Your best friend has really negative feelings about condoms. Every time you talk about condoms, this person has something negative to say about them. You decide that you will make a positive comment about condoms for every negative one that is made. What do you reply to each of the following:*

Negative comment:

"Condoms cost too much."
"It's too hard to get condoms."
"Condoms break. So why use them?"
"Condoms don't feel good."
"Condoms spoil the mood."

Positive reply:

The teacher should use her/his judgement as to correct responses.

(see Unit 3 / Student activity 2 for positive condom comments)

NEEDS ANALYSIS FOR THE TEACHER TRAINING PROGRAMME

You will be taking part in a teacher training programme on HIV/AIDS/STD. The results of this survey will be used in designing the training programme. Thank you for your collaboration.

Read each item and tick one of the three boxes.

Knowledge of HIV and AIDS

	True	Don't know	False
1. Many people who are infected with HIV can look and feel healthy.			
2. AIDS can be cured.			
3. Males who are infected with HIV can give it to another person through their semen.			
4. People who are infected with HIV can give it to another person through their blood.			
5. A mother can pass HIV to her unborn child.			
6. People can reduce their chances of becoming infected with HIV by using a latex condom during sexual intercourse.			
7. A person can become infected with HIV by being bitten by an insect such as a mosquito.			
8. A person can become infected with HIV by donating (giving) blood.			
9. People who are careful to have sexual intercourse only with healthy-looking partners won't become infected with HIV.			
10. People can be infected with HIV and not know they have it.			

Scoring procedure - knowledge:

One point is given for each correct answer, and 0 points for "don't know" and an incorrect response.

Scoring key
True: 1, 3, 4, 5, 6, 10.
False: 2, 7, 8, 9.

An item-by-item analysis of responses can help identify those content areas that may require special instruction.

Attitudes towards people with HIV or AIDS

	True	Don't know	False
1. I wouldn't mind having a student with HIV in my classroom.			
2. A student who is infected with HIV should be able to eat lunch with other students.			
3. I would avoid a student whose family member had AIDS.			
4. I would work with another teacher who was infected with HIV.			
5. Students infected with HIV should be separated from other students.			
6. Students who are infected with HIV should not play sports with other students.			
7. I would feel uncomfortable about giving individual help to a student infected with HIV.			
8. People who have AIDS should not be allowed to work in places that handle food.			
9. If I thought a teacher was infected with HIV, I would be afraid to shake hands with that teacher.			
10. I would feel comfortable hugging a friend who has AIDS.			

Scoring procedures - attitudes

To obtain a total score for each educator, add the point values of the responses. The higher the total score, the higher the acceptance of persons with HIV or AIDS. The lower the total score, the lower the acceptance of persons with HIV or AIDS (the minimum score is 10, the maximum score is 50).

The following scale should be used to score the items.

For items: 1, 2, 4,10
Agree = 5
Not Sure = 3
Disagree = 1

For items: 3, 5, 6, 7, 8, 9
Agree = 1
Not Sure = 3
Disagree = 5

Comfort with sensitive topics

How comfortable are you in discussing the following topics with students?

	Very comfartable	Somewhat comfortable	Not at all comfortable
1. How HIV is transmitted			
2. Sexual intercourse			
3. AIDS			
4. Condom use			
5. Delaying sex			
6. Male sexual organs			
7. Female sexual organs			
8. Injecting drug use			
9. Varieties of sexual behaviour			
10. Tolerance towards people with AIDS			

Scoring procedures - comfort

A high score on each item indicates a high degree of comfort and a low score indicates a low degree of comfort. The following scale should be used to score items (the minimum score is 10, the maximum score is 50).

Very comfortable: 5 points
Somewhat comfortable: 3 points
Not at all comfortable: 1 point

THREE-DAY TEACHER TRAINING AGENDA

Three-day training agenda for teachers of the HIV/AIDS/STD education workshop

1 Day

A. *Opening*

B. *Overview of the AIDS/STD situation in country*
- Prevalence of HIV/AIDS, by age/sex
- Prevalence of STD, by age/sex
- Prevention programmes

C. *Transmission and prevention of HIV/STD*
- Presentation
- Questions/Answers

D. *Young people and sexuality*
- Ages at first intercourse
- Changing patterns of marriage and sexual relations
- STD and early pregnancy in young people

E. *Adults and young people's sexuality*
- Parents' attitudes
- Teachers' attitudes

- Education about sex-related issues in school (contraception, prevention of STD)

F. *Teachers' perceptions on HIV/AIDS*
- Attitudes towards people with HIV/AIDS
- Teachers and students with HIV in the school

G. *Presentation of results of the Needs Analysis for Teachers*

H. *Teaching methods in HIV/AIDS/STD Education*

---

2 Day

A. *Introduction*
- Warm-up activities

B. *Overview of programme*
- Objectives
- Conceptual framework
- The fourunits

C. *The teacher's guide*
- Explanation of part l/Introductory information
- Explanation of part 2/Guides to the student activities

D. *Basic knowledge of HIV/AIDS/STD Unit 1*
- Overview of unit
- Explanation and demonstration of activities from Unit I

E. *Responsible behaviour: delaying sex Unit 2*
- Overview of unit
- Explanation and demonstration of activities from Unit 2

F. *The peer leader programme*
- Function and selection of peer leaders
- Objectives of the training programme for peer leaders
- Explanation of the peer leader guide

---

3 Day

A. *Review of day 2*
- Overview of day 2
- Questions

B. *Responsible behaviour - protected sex Unit 3*
- Overview of the unit
- Explanation and demonstration of activities from Unit 3

C. *Participation of parents and families*
- Why involve parents and family members
- Introduction to the parent materials
- Dealing with parent questions

D. *Care and support for people with HIV/ AIDS - Unit 4*
- Overview of the unit
- Explanation and demonstration of activities from Unit 4

E. *Evaluation of students*
- Purposes of evaluating students
- The test(s) for assessing students

F. *How to deal with students who disclose personal problems with HIV/AIDS/ STD*

TEACHER SATISFACTION WITH TRAINING WORKSHOP

1. Please rate the following workshop topics on the quality of their presentation in the workshop.

	QUALITY Excellent	Satisfactory	Poor
a. Discussion of sensitive topics.			
b. Activities in the knowledge of HIV/AIDS/STD unit.			
c. Activities in the delaying sex unit			
d. Activities in the protected sex unit			
e. Activities in the care and support unit			
f. Description of the Teachers' guide			
g. Explanation of the use of peer leaders			
h. Explanation of parents' participation			
i. Explanation of the student evaluation component			

2. Please rate the quality of the following:

	QUALITY Excellent	Satisfactory	Poor
a. Participant sessions			
b. Role-plays			
c. Demonstrations			
d. Quality of facilitators			

3. Which aspect of the training workshop was the most useful to you?
4. Which aspect of the training workshop was the least useful to you?
5. What additional topics should have been included in the training workshop?
6. What topics should have been treated in more depth in the training workshop?
7. What other comments do you have about the training workshop, and what changes need to be made?

C

Programme Evaluation Instruments

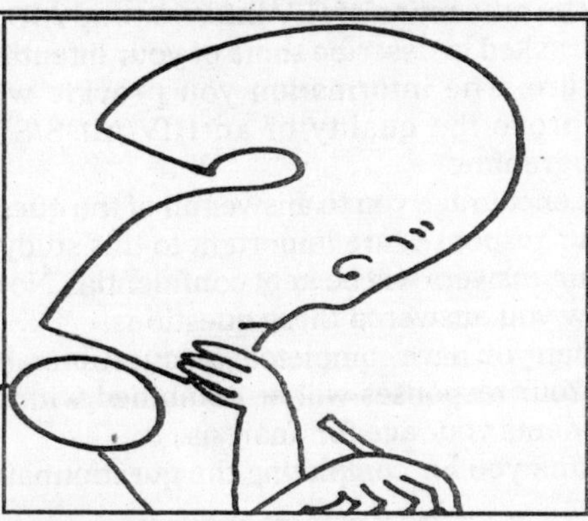

MODEL PRE-POST TEST

Instructions to teachers

1. Tell the students that the questionnaire asks for personal answers so it is important to work alone and not communicate with anyone.
2. Hand out the questionnaires and ask the students to turn the questionnaires over (upside-down) and not begin until instructed to do so.
3. Remind students that they are not to write their names on the questionnaires. Explain that the questionnaire is confidential (no one will know who has given the answers). The answers will only be seen by researchers.
4. Tell the students that this is not a test on which they will be graded.

5. Read the instructions aloud to the students.
6. Tell the students that you will not walk around the room during the test, so that their answers will be complete]y private.
7. Ask if students have any questions about the questionnaire. Answer these questions, then ask them to complete the questionnaire.
8. Because some of the students may believe that some of the false statements are, in fact, true, it is important to discuss the correct answers with students as soon as possible following the questionnaire's completion and collection.

Instructions to students

1. The purpose of this questionnaire is to obtain information about your knowledge, attitudes and skills with respect to the prevention of HIV infection and AIDS. As well, you are asked to describe some of your intentions in the near future. The information you provide will be used to improve the quality of an HIV/AIDS/STD education programme.
2. We encourage you to answer all of the questions because your responses are important to this study.
3. Your answers will be kept confidential. No one will know how you answered these questions.
4. When you have completed the questionnaire, do not sign it. Your responses will be combined with those of other students your age for analysis.
5. Thank you for completing the questionnaire.

Age	Sex	Date

Your knowledge

Instructions: Read each question. Tick the answer that fits best. Some of these questions use the words "having sex." This means sexual intercourse.

	True	Don't know	False
1. STD can be cured, but there is no cure for AIDS.			
2. One can recognize a person infected with HIV by how she/he looks.			
3. HIV is transmitted through semen and vaginal fluids and blood.			

	True	Don't know	False
4. You can get HIV if you have sex once, without a condom.			
5. You can get HIV by hugging or touching a person who has HIV or AIDS.			
6. A person can get HIV by giving (donating) blood.			
7. The more sexual partners a person has, the greater the chance of getting infected with HIV or a sexually transmitted disease.			
8. People who choose only healthy-looking partners won't get infected with HIV.			
9. There are drugs available that can help prolong the life of a person with AIDS.			
10. A good reason to delay sexual intercourse is the risk of HIV, STD and pregnancy.			
11. Assertive people get their way by overpowering others.			
12. If a person tries to get you to do something you don't want to do, you should either refuse, delay, or bargain with that person.			
13. Condoms protect a person from HIV and STD if they are used correctly every time one has sexual intercourse.			
14. A condom can be safely reused			
15. "No condom, no sex" is a good rule to protect yourself from HIV and STD.			
16. It is important to keep condoms in a warm, moist place, before use.			
17. A person with HIV who is not allowed to attend school is an example of discrimination.			
18. A person can get HIV from living in the same home with a person who has HIV or AIDS.			
19. A person with AIDS who is sweating, vomiting and has diarrhoea needs extra food.			

Scoring procedures for knowledge items

Each correct answer receives one point.

— If the correct answer was false, a student would receive one point for answering, "false".

— If the correct answer was true, a student would receive one point for answering, "true".

— Don't know scores count 0 points, but the number of "don't know" responses should be recorded for each question.

Percentage of students correct, wrong, and "don't know" should be calculated. These scores when compared to the control group will provide you with information on the achievement of your knowledge objectives.

Scoring key

True:1, 3, 4, 7, 9, 10, 12, 13, 15, 17
False:2.5.6.8. 11. 14, 16, 18, 19

Your attitudes

Instructions: Read each statement, and circle A if you agree, circle NS if you are not sure, or circle D if you disagree.

		Agree	Not Sure	Disagree
1.	Young people should realize that if they do not protect them-selves, they could get infected with HIV.	A	NS	D
2.	It is alright to have sex without a condom, because your chance of getting infected with HIV is very low.	A	NS	D
3.	It is alright not to have sex while you are a teenager.	A	NS	D
4.	It is alright for young people to have sex without a condom if they know each other well.	A	NS	D
5.	If people think they might have sex with a partner, they should carry a condom with them.	A	NS	D
6.	A young person can inject drugs once in a while without the risk of getting infected with HIV.	A	NS	D
7.	It would be alright with me to be in the same classroom with someone who has AIDS.	A	NS	D
8.	People who have AIDS should be forced to live far away from other people.	A	NS	D
9.	I would feel comfortable hugging a close friend who had AIDS.	A	NS	D
10.	It is alright to say "no" to friends when they want me to do things I do not want to do.	A	NS	D
11.	If your boy/girlfriend wants you to have sex, it is better to agree rather than to lose him/her.	A	NS	D

Scoring procedures for attitude items

Attitudes about	*Questions*	*Scoring key*
Peer pressure	10	A=3, NS=2,D=1
Abstinence/delaying	3	A=3, NS=2,D=1
	11	A=l, NS=2,D=3
Condoms	4	A=l, NS=2,D=3
	5	A=3, NS=2,D=1
Drugs	6	A=1, NS=2,D=3
Threat of HIV	I	A=3, NS=2,D=1
	2	A=l, NS=2,D=3
People with AIDS	7	A=3, NS=2,D=1
	8	A=l, NS=2,D=3
Caring for someone with AIDS	9	A=3, NS=2,D=1

Higher scores on each item reflect positive attitudes.

Overall attitude scores and scores on each attitude will be analyzed and the results from experimental and control groups, compared.

Your skills

Instructions: Try to imagine yourself in the story. Circle how confident you feel: very, some what, not at all.

1. You like your boy/girlfriend very much. He/she wants to have sex with you, but you don't. How confident are you that you could refuse and still remain friends?	Very confident	Somewhat confident	Not at all confident
2. You have been going out with someone and you have been having sex without condoms. You have heard that using a condom is a good way to keep from getting infected with HIV. Your partner does not like condoms. You do not want to have sex anymore without a condom. How confident are you that you could refuse?	Very confident	Somewhat confident	Not at all confident
3. You have bought condoms to protect you and your partner when you have sex. You really want to use condoms. confident are you in being able to use the condom properly?	Very confident	Somewhat confident	Not at all confident

Scoring procedures for skill items

Higher scores reflect better skills.

Very confident = 3

Somewhat confident = 2
Not at all confident = 1

These scores will be analyzed by refusal skills (items 1 and 2), and condom skills (item 3); they could also be accumulated to obtain an overall skill score, and compared with the control group.

Your intentions

Instructions: Read each statement and circle the one that is most true for you.

In the next six months...

1	A)	I do not intend to inject drugs
	B)	I might use injecting drugs
2	A)	I do not intend to have sex
	B)	I might have sex
	C)	I might have sex with two or more people

If you circled B or C in statement 2, please answer the following

In the next six months...

3	A)	I will use condoms with my sexual partners
	B)	It is unlikely that I will use condoms with my sexual partners
	C)	I will not have sex without a condom

Scoring procedures for behavioural intentions

Calculate the percentage of students who choose each response. Higher scores reflect safer behavioural intentions.

Question 1: A= 2, B= O
Question 2: A= 2, B= O, C= O
Question 3: A= 1, B= O, C= 1

When compared with control groups, effective programmes lead to increased percentages of students moving towards low risk behaviour.

ADDITIONAL QUESTIONS FOR PRE-POST TEST

Your knowledge

Questions	T = True F = False
1. People with AIDS die from serious illnesses.	T
2. Gonorrhoea is an example of a sexually transmitted disease.	T

3. HIV may be passed from a mother to her unborn child. T
4. You may get HIV from sharing unsterilized needles for drugs, tattooing, and ear or nose piercing. T
5. You may get HIV by drinking from the same glass that a person with AIDS has used. T
6. You may get HIV by eating food prepared by someone who has HIV or AIDS. F
7. The best method of protection against HIV and STD is to abstain from sexual intercourse. F
8. Some methods of protection against HIV or STD are better than others. T
9. The birth control pill protects from HIV or STD. T
10. There is no way to find out if you are infected with HIV. F
11. AIDS can be cured if you are given medicines early enough. F
12. Vaseline is a good lubricant to use with a condom. T
13. Lubricated condoms break more often than those that are not lubricated. F
14. If a condom slips off the penis, into the female vagina, she will become sick. T
15. It is safe to have sex just once without a condom. T
16. Being compassionate to a person with AIDS is dangerous because there is a good chance you will become infected with HIV. T
17. People with AIDS should be encouraged to do as much as they can for themselves. F
18. People with AIDS, who are upset, should be encouraged to cry or be angry. F
23. You may get HIV from sharing injecting needles and syringes for use of drugs. T
24. You may get HIV by cutting your skin with an unsterilized razor blade or other sharp instrument that was used by someone else. F
25. You may get HIV from toilet seats. F
26. You may get HIV from wearing clothes that have been worn by another person with HIV. T
27. A person who has an STD is at greater risk of getting HIV. F
28. There is evidence that HIV can be spread by some types of insects. T
29. There is no way to kill HIV on a drug injecting needle or syringe. F
30. Once you are infected with HIV, you are infected for life. T
31. Only a person who is sick with AIDS can give HIV to others. F

32. A person can have a negative test for HIV and still be infected with HIV. T
33. People infected with HIV are usually very thin and sickly. F
34. The time from being infected with HIV to getting AIDS can be as short as 6 months to as long as 10 years or more. T
35. There are drugs available that can help prolong the life of a person with AIDS. T
36. A reason to get tested for HIV is so that you will not infect others. T
37. The test for HIV looks for HIV antibodies. T
38. Men and women often have very different thoughts about sexual intercourse. T

Attitudes

Instructions: Read each statement, and circle A if you agree, circle NS if you are not sure, or circle D if you disagree.

		Agree	Not Sure	Disagree
1.	It is a good idea for teenagers to delay having sex until they are older or married.	A	NS	D
2.	A person does not have to feel bad about delaying or refusing sex.	A	NS	D
3.	If I chose to, I could easily abstain from having sexual intercourse.	A	NS	D
4.	I would be too embarrassed to use a condom.	A	NS	D
5.	I would be too embarrassed to buy a condom.	A	NS	D
6.	Using shared instruments (razors, knives) to cut the skin is alright if you do it only once or twice.	A	NS	D
7.	A person who has AIDS should not be allowed to eat lunch with other students.	A	NS	D
8.	I would stay away from someone in my class who had someone in their family with AIDS.	A	NS	D
9.	People who have AIDS are getting what they deserve.	A	NS	D
10.	I would be comfortable caring for someone who had AIDS.	A	NS	D
11.	I feel we should do more to help people who have AIDS.	A	NS	D
12.	I don't like it when friends talk me into doing things I know are dangerous.	A	NS	D

13.	I think it is alright to accept gifts or presents from people I do not know.	A	NS	D
14.	I would get tested if I thought I might have HIV.	A	NS	D
15.	If I wanted, I would be able to be affectionate without having sexual intercourse.	A	NS	D
16.	I am an assertive person.	A	NS	D
17.	I try to support my friends when they do something that is healthy.	A	NS	D
18.	If I were using drug injecting needles I would clean them with bleach.	A	NS	D

Scoring procedure for attitude items

Question	Scoring key	Question	Scoring key
1	A=3, NS=2,D=1	10	A=3, NS=2,D=1
2	A=3, NS=2,D=1	11	A=3, NS=2,D=1
3	A=3, NS=2,D=1	12	A=3, NS=2,D=1
4	A=l, NS=2,D=3	13	A=l, NS=2,D=3
5	A=l, NS=2,D=3	14	A=3, NS=2,D=1
6	A=1, NS=2,D=3	15	A=3, NS=2,D=1
7	A=l, NS=2,D=3	16	A=3, NS=2,D=1
8	A=l, NS=2,D=3	17	A=3, NS=2,D=1
9	A=l, NS=2,D=3	18	A=3, NS=2,D=1

Higher scores on each item reflect positive attitudes.

Overall attitude scores and scores on each attitude will be analyzed and the results from experimental and control groups, compared.

Skills

1. You are at a celebration where some of your friends are drinking alcohol. They want you to join them and are pressuring you to do so. If you did not want to join your friends in drinking, how confident are you that you could refuse?	Very confident	Somewhat confident	Not at all confident
2. It is a Sunday afternoon, and you have been putting off your chores and homework all weekend. You have got enough work to fill the rest of the day. Your best friend calls to invite you to go to a movie that you have both been wanting to see. If you did not want to go with your friend, how confident are you that you could refuse?	Very confident	Somewhat confident	Not at all confident

3. You are with a group of friends. One friend brings equipment to inject drugs. Some of your friends join in and seem to be having a great time. They urge you to join them. You know that sharing needles to inject drugs is an easy way to get infected with HIV. If you did not want to join your friends in injecting drugs, how confident are you that you could refuse?	Very confident	Somewhat confident	Not at all confident
4. You find yourself alone in a deserted area with a boy you thought was quite nice. Suddenly he is sayir g things and touching you in a way that makes you feel very uncomfortable. He begins to pressure you to have sex with him. If you do not want to have sex with him, how confident are you that you could refuse and get out of the situation?	Very confident	Somewhat confident	Not at all confident
5. You have been going with a boy for some time now and you have decided to have sex with him. One evening, when the two of you are alone, the opportunity for sex occurs. You even have a condom because you do not want to get HIV. However, your boyfriend becomes very upset and angry at you for thinking that he would use a condom. If you defInitely do not want to have sex without a condom, how confident are you that you could refuse?	Very confident	Somewhat confident	Not at all confident
6. You have selected a package of condoms and now must pay for them. As you get near the counter to pay for them, you notice the shop assistant is someone of the opposite sex. If you realiy wanted those condoms, how confident are you that you would still be able to buy them?	Very confident	Somewhat confident	Not at all confident
7. You do not have money to buy a condom but you have heard that you can get them free at the local health centre. If you wanted to use a condom, how confident would you be to go to the health centre for condoms?	Very confident	Somewhat confident	Not at all confident

Teacher feedback form

1. School / district: ____________________
2. Grade level: ____________________
3. Number of students in class: ____________________
4. Sex of students: ____________________
5. Sex of teacher: ____________________

Please fill in this form for Activity Number...

Answer the following questions by ticking Yes or No, and add comment:

	Yes	No
1. Was the activity clearly described?		
2. Was the activity relevant to students?		
3. Was the language appropriate?		
4. Were the pictures/graphics appropriate?		
5. Was students' participation satisfactory?		
6. Was students' learning satisfactory?		
7. Did students find the activity easy? (indicate which parts were found difficult)		
8. Was class management easy for you?		
9. (if applicable) Were peer leaders helpful?		
10. Was the Teachers' Guide useful for this activity?		
11. Did the Teachers' Guide include all that was needed to carry out the activity?		
12. Was it difficult for you to deal with the topics addressed in the activity? If so, which ones?		

13. My suggestions for improvement of this activity are:
____
____
____
____
____

14. My suggestions for improvement of the Teachers' Guide on this activity are:
____
____
____
____

15. How much classroom time was spent on this activity? (in minutes) [|]

TEACHER INTERVIEW

Notes to interviewer

1. Each question in the interview should be asked so that the teacher has a chance to expand or explain their answer.
2. Wait for the teacher's responses without influencing the answer.
3. Even though you will ask to tape record the interview, enter the responses as you hear them (i.e. tick the appropriate response choice) and record a few words that will help you elaborate or clarify an answer.
4. Expand or clarify answers from the tape recorder so that someone else can interpret them.
5. You will be asking these questions with reference to one class. If the teacher has taught the programme to more than one class, ask for reference to be made primarily to the latest class taught.

Teacher interview

A) Background information

1. Date of interview Day [ ] Month [ ] Year [ ]
2. School/District ____________________
3. Sex (of teacher) Male [ ] Female [ ]
4. Sex (of students) Male [ ] Female [ ] Total [ ]
5. Number of hours in programme [ ] Hours
6. How many years have you been teaching?
   a) in total: [|]

b) this grade level/age: ☐☐

c) area/subject: ☐☐

7. a) Do you have any training in teaching sexuality or AIDS, other than the teacher workshop you attended? Yes ☐ No ☐

b) If yes, specify what the training was: ____________

B) Teacher attitudes about the programme

8.a) Would you want to teach this programme on HIV/AIDS/STD again?

Yes	No	only in part
☐	☐	☐

b) If not the whole programme, which parts would you want to teach? *[Tick one or more boxes, as appropriate]*

Unit 1 ☐	Unit 3 ☐
Unit 2 ☐	Unit 4 ☐

9. Rate the parts of the programme that you were most and least comfortable with

	Most	Least		Most	Least
The activities in unit 1:	☐	☐	The peer leader help:	☐	☐
The activities in unit 2:	☐	☐	Parent involvement:	☐	☐
The activities in unit 3:	☐	☐	Assertiveness skills:	☐	☐
The activities in unit 4:	☐	☐	Condom skills:	☐	☐

Other: ____________

C) The students

10. What was the age range of students in your class? ☐☐ to ☐

11. Generally, how was the reading level of the activities for most of your students?

Too high	Alright	Too low
☐	☐	☐

12. How would you describe the students' overall involvement in the programme's activities?

High	Moderate	Too low
☐	☐	☐

D) The parents

13. a) Did you receive any positive comments from the parents about the programme? Yes ☐ No ☐

b) If yes, how many?: ____________

c) If yes, give an example: ____________

14. How did you involve parents? *[Tick one or more boxes, as appropriate]*

parent meeting	☐	letter to parents	☐
student activities at home	☐	leaflet	☐
parent/student interview	☐	drama, exhibition	☐
other			

E) The peer leaders

15. Did you use peer leaders to help you with the programme?

Yes ☐ No ☐

16. How much time did you spend training the peer leaders?

☐☐ Hours

17. How effective were the peer leaders in the programme?

Very effective ☐

Moderately effective ☐

Not effective ☐

18. a) Would you recommend any changes to the peer leader part of the programme?

Yes ☐ No ☐

b) If yes, what changes? ____________

____

____

____

____

19. To what extent did the peer leaders help the students?

Greatly ☐ Somewhat ☐ Little ☐ Not at all ☐

20. How did the peer leaders help in classroom management?

____

____

____

____

F) Teacher training

21. a) How do you feel about the teacher training programme now that you have finished the programme?

Very satisfied	Satisfied	Dissatisfied	Very dissatisfied
☐	☐	☐	☐

b) If dissatisfied, why?

____

____

____

22. Was the training long enough?

Too short	Alright	Too long
☐	☐	☐

23. How well did the training prepare you for teaching the programme?

Very well	Quite well
☐	☐
Didnotneed	Not well enough the training
☐	☐

24. Do you have anything to add about the teacher training?

____

____

G) Evaluation of students

25. a) Did you use the evaluation materials to give the students a grade or mark?

Yes	No
☐	☐

b) If yes, which ones? *[Tick one or more boxes, as appropriate]* true-false questions ☐ short answer questions ☐

skill questions ☐ life situation questions ☐

26. a) Are there changes you would like to make to the evaluation questions?

Yes ☐ No ☐

b) If yes, what changes? ______________________________

____

____

H) Teaching methods

27. Were you able to make copies of the activity sheets for each student?

Yes ☐ No ☐

28. Did you write the activities on the blackboard?

All ☐ Most ☐ Some ☐ None ☐

29. Did you read the activities to the students?

All ☐ Most ☐ Some ☐ None ☐

30. Did you use small groups for the activities?

Yes ☐ No ☐

31. a) Did you have trouble carrying out the activities?

Yes ☐ Some ☐ No ☐

b) If yes, please tell us what the difficulties were:

____

____

____

____

32. Do you have any recommendations that would make it easier for you to use the activities?

I) Sensitive issues

33. a) Did sensitive issues come up while teaching the programme?

Yes ☐ No ☐

b) If yes, what were they? ______________________________

c) Did the teacher's guide help you to deal with these issues?

Yes ☐ No ☐

d) If no, what other help would you like to see in the guide about sensitive issues?

J) Personal changes/issues

34. Did the programme affect you in any way?

Yes ☐ No ☐ Don't know ☐

If yes in what way?

35. Will you change anything about the way you teach as result of the programme?

Yes ☐ No ☐ Don't know ☐

If yes, what will you change?

CHECKLIST FOR STUDENT FOCUS GROUP

A) Background

1. Date of interview: __________
2. School/district: __________
3. Teacher: __________
4. Number of students in the group: (male/female) __________

B) Activities

1. Speaking generally: What did you think of the HIV/AIDS/STD Programme activities? What did you like and/or dislike?

2. Do you remember the four steps to an assertive message? What are they?

3. How did you find practising how to deliver an assertive message?

4. How did you feel about the condom activities? What did you learn from doing them?

5. What did you think about the discrimination and compassion activities towards the end of the programme? What did you learn from them?

6. How did you feel about the parent activities (if activities were done with parents)? Was it the first time you talked about those topics with your parents or other relatives?

7. Do you think your parents learned anything about HIV/AIDS?

8. Were there any activities you really liked? If so, which ones and why?

9. a) Were there any activities you really disliked? Which ones and why?

   b) If yes, how would you change the activity to make it better ?

10. What about the situations (scenarios) within the activities - were they useful? Did you feel they were realistic/may happen to you or your friends?

11. Were you able to read and understand the language? Was it too difficult? Was it too easy?

C) Peer leaders (if used)

1. What did you think about the use of peer leaders in the programme? Were they helpful? Were they used too much/too little?

____

____

2. Were the peer leaders well chosen?

____

____

3. Would you have liked to be a peer leader? Why?

____

____

4. Would you change anything about the peer leader role to make them more useful?

____

____

D) Overall evaluation

1. Do you think you can now protect yourself from HIV/AIDS/STD? How? What about in the future?

____

____

2. Did you talk about HIV/AIDS/STD with your friends? With your boy/girlfriend? With friends who did not have such a programme? With siblings or cousins? In your church youth group?

____

____

3. Do you have any other comments to add? (e.g. - were there any aspects which really bothered you about the programme that you haven't already mentioned? Were there other aspects which you were pleased about?)

____

____

____

Parent interview

The parent interview format will depend on the type of activities planned for parent and family involvement. Choose from the questions below those you think are relevant and add others.

A) Background

1. Date of interview: ______________________________

2. School/district: ____________________

3. Teacher's name: ____________________

4. Sex of parent: ____________________

5. Sex of student: ____________________

B) Possible questions

1. How do you feel about your son/daughter learning about sex and AIDS at school?

2. Have you seen any of the materials used in the programme? Which ones?

3. Have you attended any parent meeting about the programme?

4. The HIV/AIDS/STD programme in the school focuses on learning information and skills to prevent HIV and STD. Overall, what do you think of involving parents in such a programme?

5. Has your son/daughter taken the initiative to talk to you about the HIV/AIDS/STD programme that he/she is taking/has taken in the school?

6. Have you taken the initiative to ask your son/daughter about the programme?

7. Did you use some of the suggested questions in the booklet?

8. Did you do any of the Student/Parent activities with your son/daughter? Which one(s)?

9. Who did the activities with your son/daughter? (mother; father; both; other relative, specify)

10. Were any of the other children involved in doing the activities?

11. About how much time was spent on the activities that you did with your son/daughter?

12. How did you find the activities (language, pictures, too personal, too much information, unclear ....)

13. Had you discussed sexuality with your children before the programme?

14. Had you discussed AIDS/STD with your children before the programme? With other children in your family?

15. Did you find it difficult? Why?

16. Where do you think your children learn about sexuality outside the family and school?

17. Would you recommend that other parents participate in the parent/guardian activities with their son/daughter?

18. Do you think the programme has affected your son/daughter in any way - either a positive or negative way?

19. Do you feel you learned something from this programme? What?

20. Are there changes you think should be made in the programme or do you have any comments that you would like to make?

This ends the interview. Thank you for the time you have spent with me completing this interview and for all your comments and suggestions. We hope that your son/daughter has benefited from the programme.

PEER LEADER FORM AND CHECKLIST FOR FOCUS GROUP

Notes to interviewer

1. Explain to the peer leaders that the function of this session is to obtain their perceptions of their training to be peer leaders and the experience of being a peer leader.
2. Explain that you would like them to complete the attached form before discussing the experience in the group.
3. Hand out a form to each peer leader. Give them sufficient time to finish the form. Stress that they do not have to sign the form.
4. Ask the questions in the checklist allowing an open discussion of each topic. Use appropriate probes where necessary.
5. If possible, tape the discussion. If this is not possible, record words or expressions that will aid you in transcribing important information at a later date.
6. Thank the students. Collect the completed forms.
7. Summarize pertinent comments from the interview and submit this summary and the completed forms to the programme evaluator.

Peer leader survey

A) Background information

Day Month Year

1. Date of interview: ☐☐ ☐☐ ☐

2. School/District: ____________________________

3. Sex: Male ☐ Female ☐

4. Age: ☐☐ Years

B) Peer leader training

5. Did you receive any training to be a peer leader? *[If no, skip to 9]*

Yes ☐ No ☐

6. What did you find most interesting in your training?

____

____

7. a) Do you think the training helped you to be a better peer leader?

Yes ☐ No ☐ Don't know ☐

b) If yes, what specific aspects were most helpful?

____

____

c) If no, what kinds of things would have helped you?

____

____

____

8. Please evaluate the following aspects of the training by ticking the appropriate box.

	Good	Fair	Poor
The peer leader manual or materials	☐	☐	☐
The instructor(s) that conducted the training	☐	☐	☐
The amount of time given to training	☐	☐	☐
The skills you learned in the workshop	☐	☐	☐

C) The peer leader experience

9. Please evaluate the following aspects of your peer leader experience by ticking the appropriate box.

	Good	Fair	Poor
My contribution to discussion	☐	☐	☐
My help to the teacher	☐	☐	☐
My listening to others	☐	☐	☐
My ability to give support and help to students	☐	☐	☐
My ability to write activities on the blackboard	☐	☐	☐
My ability to read parts of activities	☐	☐	☐
Help you received from your teacher	☐	☐	☐
Reactions of your peers during the activity	☐	☐	☐
Reactions of your peers after class.	☐	☐	☐

10. a) Would you be a peer leader again if you were asked?

Yes	No	Don't know
☐	☐	☐

b) Why? ______________________________

____

____

____

Checklist for group discussion

1. What aspects of being a peer leader bothered you?

____

____

2. What aspects did you like?

____

____

3. What did you find most difficult?

____

____

4. What changes would you like to see, if you were asked to do this task again?

____

____

5. How would you improve the training you received?

____

____

____

SCHOOL DIRECTOR'S INTERVIEW

Notes to interviewer

Each question should be asked in an open-ended way. Wait for the responses and only use the probes or response choices if the director gives no response or the question is not understood.

Record responses as you hear them (i.e. - tick the appropriate response) and write down the main points of what was said when elaboration is needed. Note and expand the explanation for responses where given so that someone else can interpret them.

School director's interview

A) Background

1. Date of interview

Day		Month		Year	

2. School/District:

3. Sex: Male ☐ Female ☐

B) General views of the programme

4. What are your overall impressions of the programme?

Very good	Good	Fair	Poor	Verypoor
☐	☐	☐	☐	☐

5. How enthusiastic were you about having it taughtinyourschool?

High ☐ Moderate ☐ Low ☐

6. a) How did the community, excluding students' parents, react to the implementation of the programme?

Positively ☐ Negatively ☐ Don't know ☐

b) Who reacted negatively? How did you respond?

7. What things helped the implementation of the programme?

8. What things hindered the implementation of the programme?

9. Do you think the programme was important for young people in your school?

Yes ☐ No ☐ Part of it ☐

10. Based on what you know about the programme, would you want to use this programme again next year?

Yes, in its entirety ☐

Yes, in part ☐

No ☐

11. Were there particular components of the programme that you liked or disliked?

	Liked	Neutral	Disliked
Peer leaders in the classroom	☐	☐	☐
Skills as part of the programme	☐	☐	☐
Unit on protected sex	☐	☐	☐
Basic knowledge unit	☐	☐	☐
Parent involvement	☐	☐	☐
Unit on delaying sex	☐	☐	☐
Care and support unit	☐	☐	☐
Student activities	☐	☐	☐

C) Student response

12. a) Did you receive any comments from students about the programme?

Yes ☐ No ☐

b) If yes, were they mostly positive, neutral,or negative?

Positive ☐ Neutral ☐ Negative ☐

D) Teachers' training

13. Did you find the teacher training programme useful?

Very useful ☐ Useful ☐ Not useful ☐

14. a) What was the general response of your teachers to the programme?

Most liked it ☐

Many were neutral ☐

Most disliked it ☐

b) Comments?

____

____

____

15. a) Could the programme developers improve the programme to help you and your teachers with the implementation?

Yes ☐ No ☐

b) If yes, how? ____________________

E) Parent/guardian involvement

16. a) Did you receive any positive comments from parents about the programme?

Yes ☐ No ☐

b) If yes, from how many parents? ____________________

c) What kinds of comments were made? ____________________

17. a) Did you receive any negative comments from parents about the programme?

Yes ☐ No ☐

b) If yes, from how many parents?
c)What were the comments?

18. a) Was there additional help/information you would like to have had for the parents/guardians?

Yes ☐ No ☐

b) If yes, what do you need? ____________________

F) Issues

19. Did any of the teachers come to you with problems?

Yes ☐ No ☐

20. If yes, what were the problems? ____________________

21. How was the teachers' overall response? ________________
____
____

22. Who were the teachers most in favour of the programme? (gender, age)
____
____

23. What kind of support did you get from the Ministry/ Administration?
____
____

24. Do you have any other comments to add? (e.g. Were there any aspects which really bothered you about the programme that you haven't already mentioned? Are there aspects that you were pleased about?)
____
____
____

PART-II

Students' Activities

Unit 1

Basic Knowledge on HIV/AIDS/STD

1.1. HIV/AIDS/STD

BASIC QUESTIONS AND ANSWERS

Why?

Everyone should know basic facts about HIV/AIDS/ STD (Human Immunodeficiency Virus, Acquired Immunodeficiency Syndrome, Sexually Transmitted Disease(s)).

How?

Your teacher will give you instructions on how to do this activity.

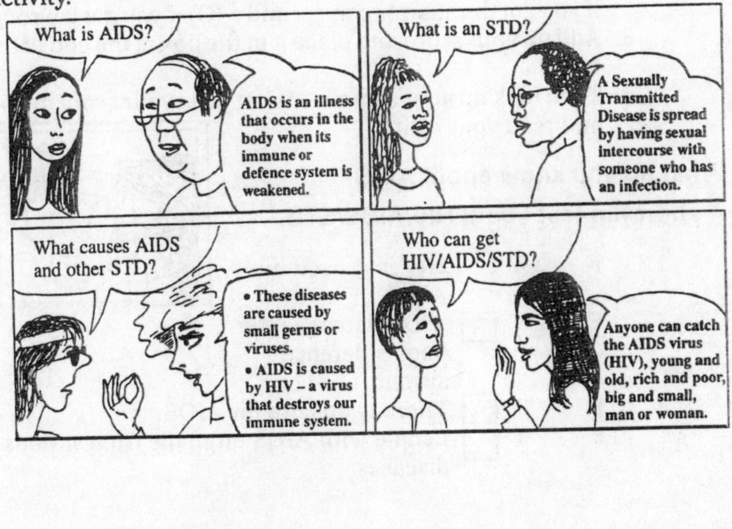

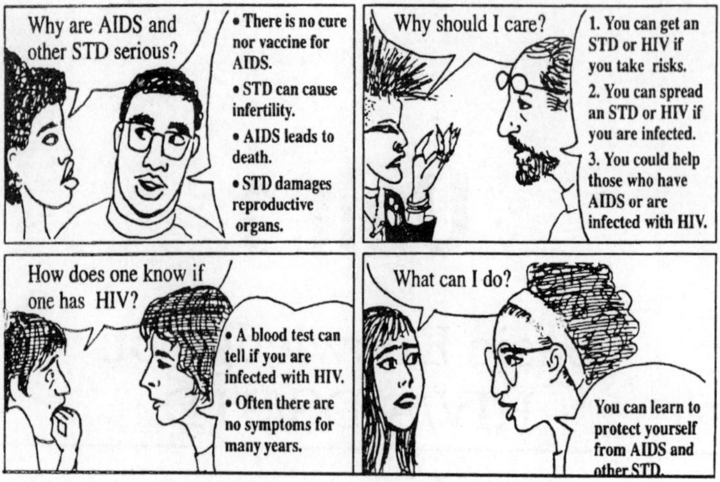
Why are AIDS and other STD serious?
• There is no cure nor vaccine for AIDS.
• STD can cause infertility.
• AIDS leads to death.
• STD damages reproductive organs.
Why should I care?
1. You can get an STD or HIV if you take risks.
2. You can spread an STD or HIV if you are infected.
3. You could help those who have AIDS or are infected with HIV.
How does one know if one has HIV?
• A blood test can tell if you are infected with HIV.
• Often there are no symptoms for many years.
What can I do?
You can learn to protect yourself from AIDS and other STD.

1.2. LOOKING INTO AIDS

Why?

You have learned something about HIV/AIDS/ STD in the first part of this lesson. This is a test to find out how much you know.

How?

1. Answer true or false to each of the statements below by placing a circle around T or F.
2. When your teacher has given your class the correct answers, place a (1) in the box to the left of each statement if you got the answer correct and a (O) if you got it wrong.
3. Add up your score and place it in the box at the end of the test.
4. Then look up your score in "What does your score mean" and read your rating.

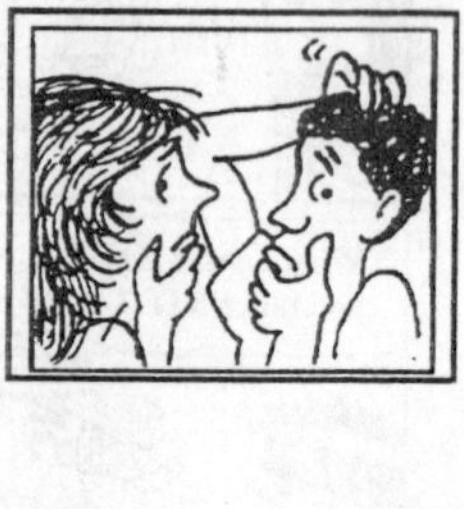

What do you know about AIDS

A short fun test about HIV/AIDS/STD

1	F	T	☐	HIV is caused by AIDS.
2	F	T	☐	AIDS damages the body's defence system.
3	F	T	☐	There is no cure for AIDS.
4	F	T	☐	People with AIDS often die from serious diseases.

5	F	T	☐	STD means Standard Time in Daylight.
6	F	T	☐	A person can have HIV or an STD and have no symptoms (not know it).
7	F	T	☐	There is no way you can protect yourself from AIDS and STD.
8	F	T	☐	An example of an STD is gonorrhoea.
9	F	T	☐	It is difficult for women to get AIDS.
10	F	T	☐	If you are strong and healthy you can t get HIV/AIDS/STD.
				Total

What does your score mean

10	8 - 9	5 - 7	3 - 4	1 - 2
Genius Expert! You can teach the class!	Good ! You are on the way to being an AIDS expert!	Well done, but you may want to look at the information again!	Review the information. You don't want to catch AIDS or STD!	Lucky for you that this is just a test! You'll do better next time!

1.3. HIV, AIDS, STD

What do they mean?

Why?

This activity will help you understand the meaning of certain words, like STD, AIDS and HIV. Knowing these words will help you understand how you can protect yourself from HIV/STD.

How?

1. Read the story A.
2. From box B pick what you think are the right words for STD, AIDS, HIV and gonorrhoea, and match the correct definition with each box in C.
3. Your teacher will tell you more about each of these words.
4. Finish the sentences in "Teacher asks".

Story A

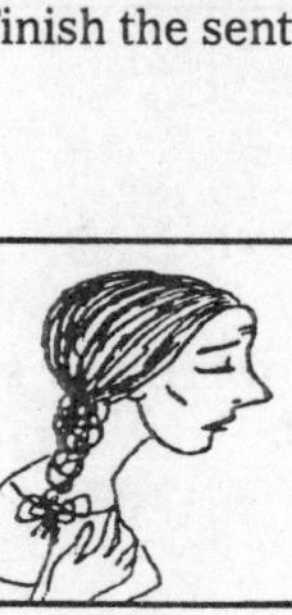

Maria wasn't feeling well. She had been losing weight and always seemed out of breath when going up stairs.

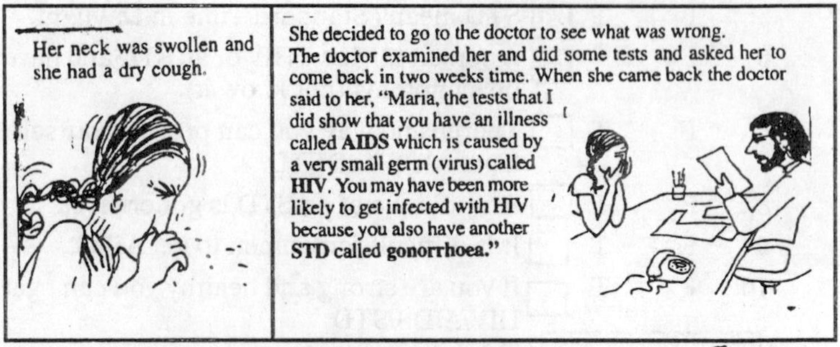

Maria wanted to know what all these words meant and how serious they were. Can you help her?

B

A Virus that weakens the defence system, allowing other diseases to enter the body.	Illnesses that occur when the body's defence system is weakened.
A type of STD that may damage reproductive organs.	Diseases that are spread by sexual contact.

C

AIDS:	HIV:
STD:	Gonorrhoea:

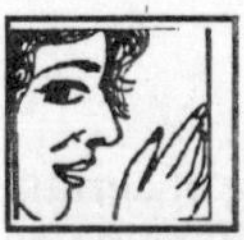

Teacher asks

Finish the sentences with your own thoughts and/ or feelings.

a) When I think of AIDS I feel: ______________________

b) HIV/AIDS is serious because: ______________________

c) STD are serious because: ______________________

d) People become infected with HIV because: ______________________

....

Tear off and place in the Dear teacher question box.

One question that I would like to ask about HIV, AIDS or STD is: ______________________

1.4. HOW A PERSON GETS HIV (the virus that causes AIDS)

Why?

It is most important to know how HIV is spread. This information can help you protect yourself.

How?

1. With your teacher read the three methods of transmission of HIV.

2. Ask any questions you might have about how HIV is spread.

Sexual intercourse

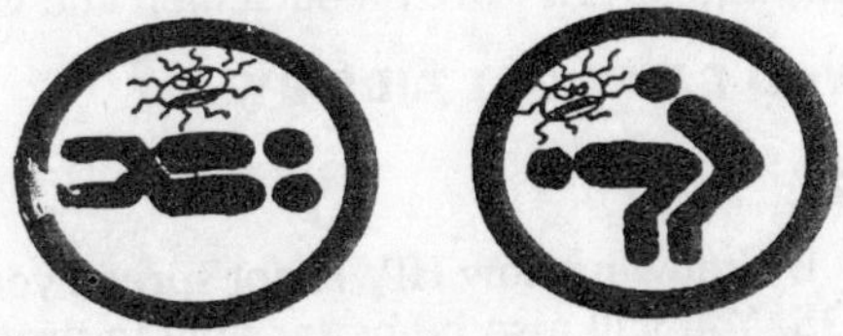

- Most people get HIV by having unprotected sexual intercourse with an infected person.
- Unprotected sexual intercourse means having vaginal or anal sex without a condom.
- HIV may also be transmitted through oral sex.

Infected blood

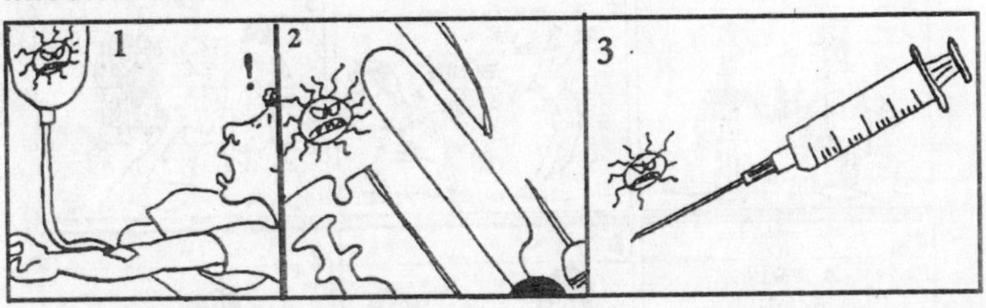

1. One can get HIV through a blood transfusion with infected blood.
2. One can get HIV by using instruments used on someone with HIV for earpiercing, tattoos or circumcision, which have not been properly cleaned.
3. One can get HIV by using needles or syringes used by someone else for injections, which have not been properly cleaned.

Infected mother to her unborn or newborn child

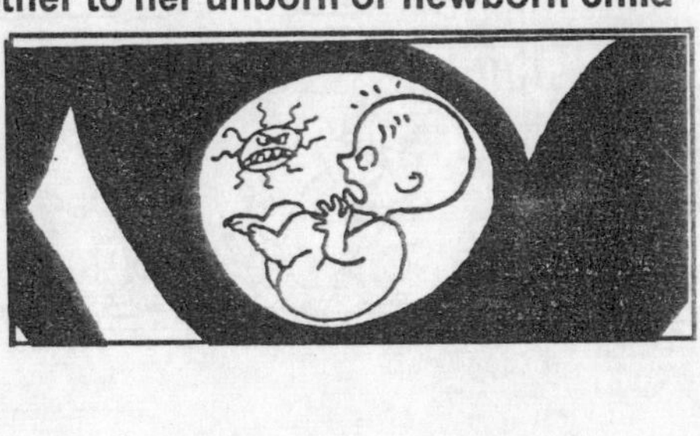

- Babies born to mothers with HIV may become infected in the womb before birth, during birth, and sometimes through breast milk.

It is not easy to get AIDS. Unlike many common diseases, HIV cannot get to us through air, food or water. The virus cannot live outside our body for long. We can only catch HIV if the body fluids of an infected person enter our body. The body fluids with a high concentration of HIV are blood semen and vaginal secretions.

1.5. YOU CAN'T GET AIDS BY...

Why?

By knowing how HIV is not spread you can reduce your fear of AIDS. You will also be better able to provide care and comfort, without fear, to someone living with AIDS.

How?

For each picture, write down what the people are doing. You will learn that HIV is not spread through any of these activities.

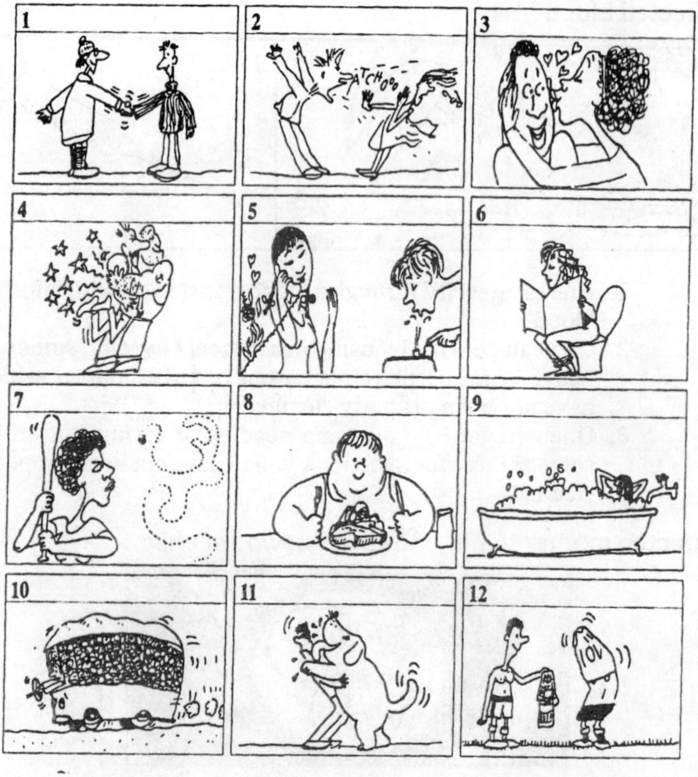

HIV does not spread through everyday contact with people who are infected with HIV. So we don't need to worry about things we do daily!

1.6. What do you believe?

A true-false test on HIV/AIDS/STD

1 T F The AIDS virus, HIV, can be spread by shaking hands.	**2** T F The AIDS virus, HIV, can be passed on to another person during sex.	**3** T F Pregnant women can pass the AIDS virus on to their unborn child.
4 T F A person can get HIV by donating blood.	**5** T F It is possible to get HIV from toilet seat.	**6** T F HIV is spread by kissing.
7 T F The AIDS virus, HIV, is carried in the blood.	**8** T F Drug users can pass on HIV to other drug users if they share needles.	**9** T F Only men can become infected by the AIDS virus, HIV.
10 T F You should avoid touching a person with AIDS.	**11** T F It is risky to use the same water fountain as a person who has AIDS.	**12** T F If you are strong and healthy you can't get HIV.
13 T F You can tell by looking at someone whether that person has the AIDS virus.	**14** T F You are safe from HIV if you cut your skin with a knife used by someone else who cut themselves.	**15** T F You are safe from HIV if you use the same condom more than once.
16 T F The risk of getting HIV/STD increases if you have many sexual partners.	**17** T F It is OK to share bedclothes and dishes with someone who has HIV/AIDS.	**18** T F It is OK to share razors with someone who has AIDS.
19 T F Young people are not at risk from HIV, the AIDS virus.	**20** T F During menstruation the risk getting HIV through unprotecte sex is higher.	

1.7. WHAT WOULD YOU DO?

Why?

You now know how the AIDS virus, HIV, is spread and how it is not spread. It is also important to know whether certain situations/activities pose high, low or no risk.

How?

1. Read each story by yourself or with your teacher.
2. Answer the questions after each story.
3. Place an "X" on the line to show the risk of getting HIV for Natombie (story 1), you (story 2) and Maria (story 3).

Story 1

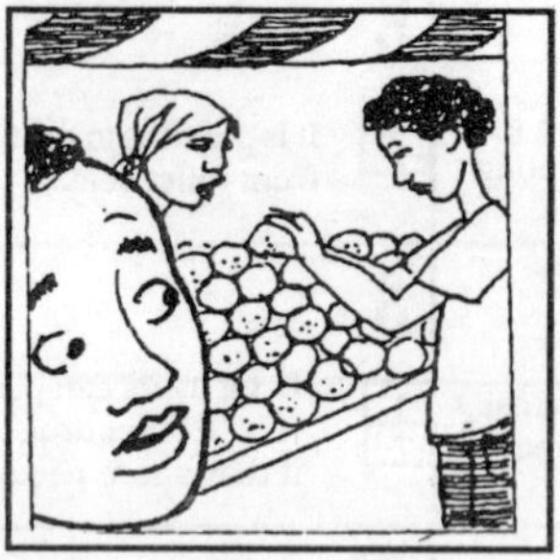

Natombie works at a fruit stand after school. He has heard that Jalondi who works there too, has AIDS. Natombie's mother has also heard this and wants him to quit his job.

a) What could Natombie tell his mother about the spread of HIV?
b) Does he need to quit his job? Why or why not?
c) What risk does Natombie have of being infected with HIV, if he works with Jalondi?

Story 2

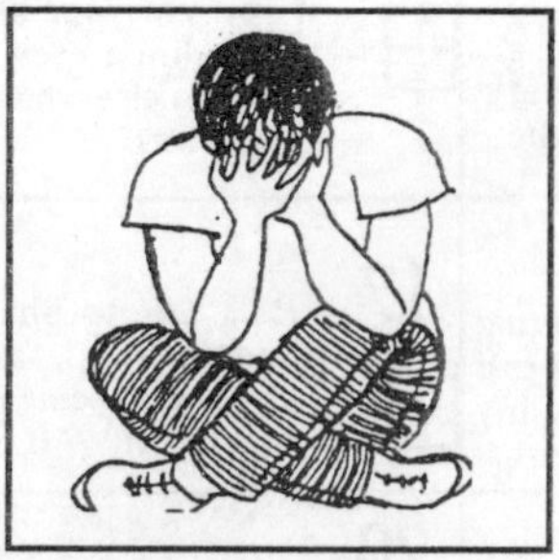

Haiwa is 15 years old and has the AIDS virus, HIV. He does not look sick but he does get tired quickly. He wants to continue going to school but wonders if he should tell anyone.

a) Do you think he should continue going to school? Why or why not?
b) Should he tell anyone? Who? Why?
c) How would you react if he told you?

d) What risk would you have of getting HIV if Haiwa sat next to you at school?

Story 3

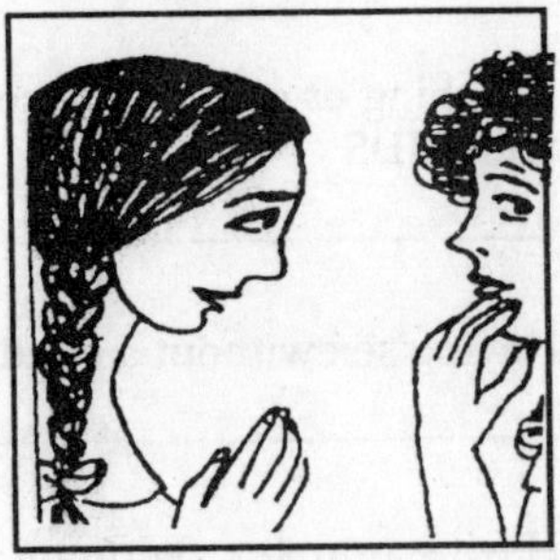

Your best friend Maria asks you what it is like to have sex. You know she goes with Roberto and you also know that Roberto has had sex with other girls.

a) What should you tell Maria? Why?

b) What risk would Maria have of getting HIV if she had sex with Roberto?

1.8. WHAT IS YOUR RISK?

Why?

Since there is no vaccine or cure for HIV/AIDS, it is important for you to know how you can get HIV. This will help you to know which things are risky and should be avoided, and which things are not.

How?

1. Read the section called "Risk levels"
2. In each of the boxes beside the activities put: NR = No Risk or LR = Low Risk or HR = High Risk

---

Risk Levels

NR No nsk of getting HIV/AIDS - there is no exchange of blood, male semen or female vaginal secretions.

LR Low risk of getting HIV/AIDS - there is a slight possibility of exchange of blood, semen or vaginal secretions.

HR High risk of getting HIV/AIDS - there is a strong possibility of exchange of blood, male semen or female vaginal secretions.

Activity	No.	
Using toilets in a public washroom.	1	☐
Touching or comforting someone living with AIDS	2	☐
Having sex without a condom	3	☐
Having oral sex (without semen in the mouth)	4	☐
Kissing (dry kissing)	5	☐
Having sex using the same condom more than once	6	☐
Sharing needles for injection drug use	7	☐
Swimming with an HIV infected person	8	☐
Sharing needles for earpiercing or tattooing	9	☐
Abstaining from sexual intercourse	10	☐
Going to school with an HIV-infected person	11	☐

Cutting the skin with a knif used by others	12	☐
Being bitten by a mosquito	13	☐
Giving blood	14	☐
Having sex using a condon properly	15	☐
Eating food prepared by an HIV-infected person	16	☐

What is your risk?

To avoid HIV/STD it is very important for you to find out your own personal risk. To do this, look at the risky activities above and consider if you have done any of them in the past. Think about where you would put an "X" on the line below to show what risk you have of getting HIV/AIDS/STD.

0 10

no risk low risk high risk

Do you think your risk of getting HIV will change as you get older? If yes, why and how?

1.9. ARE YOU AT RISK? (PART 1)

Why?

Since there is no vaccine or cure for HIV/AIDS it is important for you to know how you can get HIV. This will help you to know which things are risky and should be avoided and which are not.

How?

1. With your teacher, read and discuss "HIV can be spread by". You should be very familiar with the methods of transmission indicated below;

2. Then go over the "Risk levels" with your teacher. Each small group will be given 6 behaviours/actions to rate as: No Risk, Low Risk, High Risk, No Agreement;
3. With the others in your group, come to an agreement on how to rate each of the behaviours/actions (you may have to take a vote to decide this). For example, your group may decide that shaking hands with someone who has HIV is no risk. Put NR beside that behaviour/action.

HIV can be spread by:

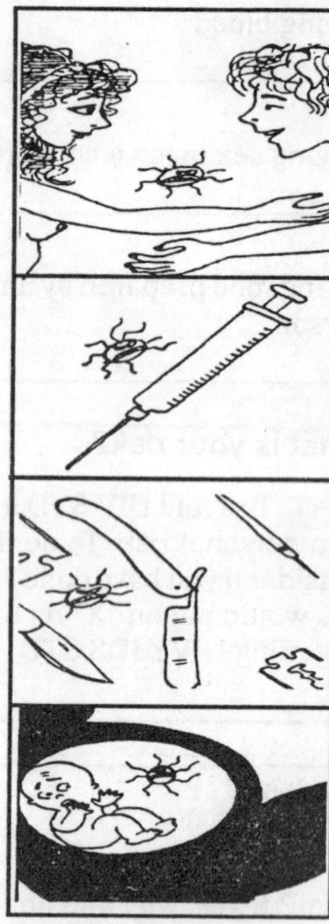

Sex

Unprotected (no condom) sexual intercourse (by vaginal, anal and possibly oral sex)

Blood

Shared injecting needles and syringes that are not clean (e.g. those used by "quack" doctors)

Shared instruments that pierce, or may pierce, the skin - razor blades, knives, needles etc.

Mother

Infected mother to baby.

Risk levels

HR ***High risk***

There is a strong possibility of exchange of blood, male semer or female vaginal secretions, e.g. sexual intercourse.

NR ***No risk***

There is no exchange of blood, male semen or female vagina secretions.

LR ***Low risk***

There is a slight possibility of exchange of blood, male semen or female vaginal secretions e.g. sex with a condom.

? *No agreement*

Your group cannot reach agreement.

Notes

STD are spread mainly by unprotected sexual intercourse and unprotected oral-genital contact. HIV can also be transmitted through a blood transfusion with infected blood.

Are you at risk?

1 Group

☐ 1. Body to body rubbing with clothes on.

☐ 2. Sharing a razor to shave legs or face.

☐ 3. Having sex with a condom - condom breaks.

☐ 4. Back rub - massage.

☐ 5. Riding on a bus with an HIV-infected person.

☐ 6. Cutting the skin with a knife used by others.

2 Group

☐ 1. Using toilets in a public washroom.

☐ 2. Sharing needles for injection drug use.

☐ 3. Being bitten by a mosquito.

☐ 4. Dry kissing.

☐ 5. Having vaginal sex without a condom.

☐ 6. Cleaning up spilled HIV infected blood without wearing gloves.

3 Group

☐ 1. Having anal sex without a condom.

☐ 2. Abstaining from sexual intercourse.

☐ 3. Sharing needles for ear-piercing.

☐ 4. Shaking hands with an HIV-infected person.

☐ 5. Having oral sex (without semen in the mouth).

☐ 6. Swimming with an HIV infected person.

Group 4

☐ 1. Sharing needles for tattooing.

☐ 2. Sharing clothes with someone who has HIV.

☐ 3. Donating blood.

☐ 4. Eating food prepared by an HIV-infected person.

☐ 5. Having sex with a number of partners - no condom.

☐ 6. Going to school with an HIV-infected person.

Group 5

☐ 1. Using public drinking fountains.

☐ 2. Giving mouth-to-mouth resuscitation if there are no sores in the mouth.

☐ 3. Having unprotected sex with an STD-infected person.

☐ 4. Playing sports with an HIV-infected person. Group

☐ 5. Sharing a needle cleaned with water.

6. Being close to an HIV-infected person who coughs or sneezes.

Group 6

1. Being bitten by an HIV infected person.
2. Wet (deep) kissing.
3. Having sex using a condom properly.
4. Sharing a towel with an HIV-infected person.
5. Touching or comforting someone living with AIDS .
6. Having sex using the same condom more than once.

Teacher asks

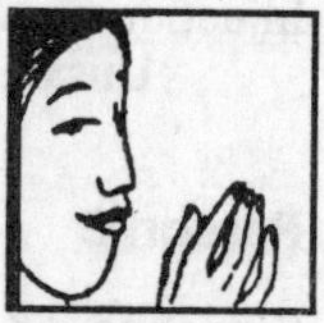

Some young people become very afraid of HIV/AIDS.

a) Why do you think they are so afraid?
b) What could be done to prevent this fear of HIV/AIDS?

1.9. ARE YOU AT RISK? (PART 2)

Why?

Often young people will take more than one risk, which means there is a greater chance of them getting HIV/STD. For example, they may inject drugs with unsterilized needles and have sex without using a condom.

How?

1. Read what persons A, B, C, D do in the descriptions below.
2. For each person, list any behaviours that would put them at risk for HIV/AIDS.
3. Finally, rate the four people according to the risks they are taking by putting the person with the safest behaviour in box 1 and the person with the least safe behaviour in box 4.

Person A

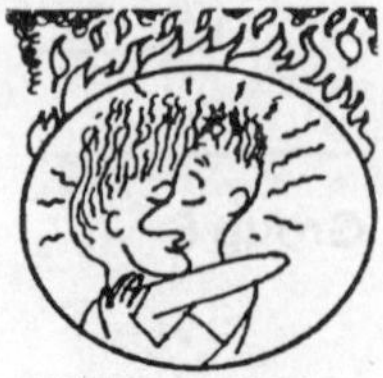

He has a relationship which involves wet kissing, hugging and touching of the genitals (sex organs).

Unsafe behaviours: ______________________________

Person B

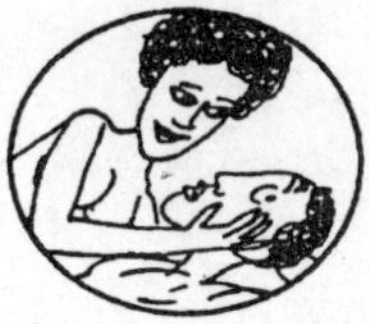

She has had sexual intercourse for the first time without a condom with her boyfriend, whom she believes has never had sex. Her boyfriend has not told her that he has had sex with a number of different people without a condom and has shared unsterilized (dirty) injection needles in the past.

Unsafe behaviours: ______________________________

Person C

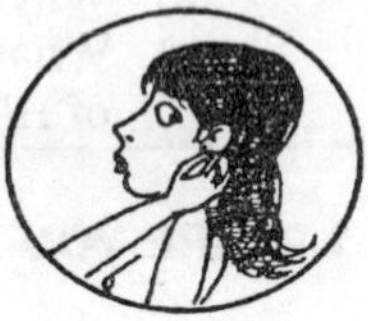

She has shared unsterilized needles for ear-piercing with her girlfriend and is having sex with a condom. Her partner has previously had sex without a condom.

Unsafe behaviours: ______________________________

Person D

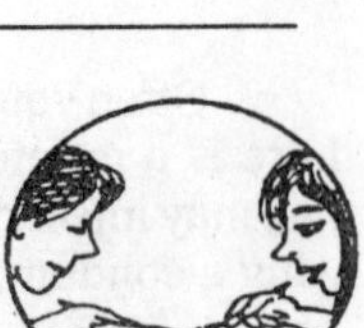

She often kisses her boyfriend (dry kissing) and lives with a brother who is HIV-positive. They share dishes and eat the same food and often hug each other.

Unsafe behaviours: ______________________________

Person with safest behaviour			Person with least safe behaviour
1	2	3	4

Teacher asks

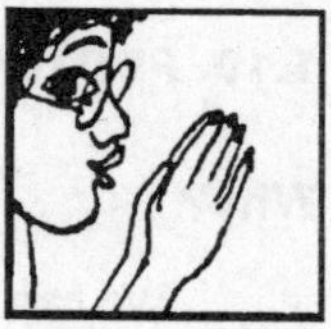

What would the person in box 4 have to do to reduce his/her chance of getting HIV/AIDS/STD?

1.9. ARE YOU AT RISK? (PART 3)

Why?

To avoid HIV/STD, it is very important for you to determine your own personal risk. To do this you need to know the number of risks you take and the risk level of each of those risk behaviours.

How?

1. On your own, estimate your personal risk of HIV/STD infection at this time in your life. Think about where you would put your "X" on the line below. Your answer is private. Do not write your answer on the line.
2. Where do you think your "X" will be 5 years from now?

On your own, estimate your personal risk of HIV/STD infection at this time in your life.

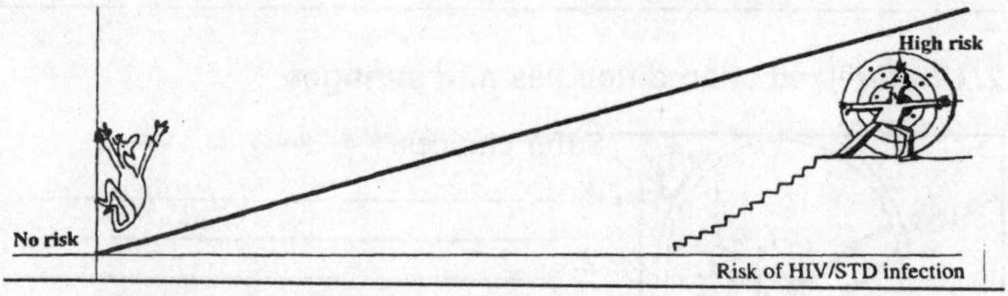

Where do you think your "X" will be 5 years from now?

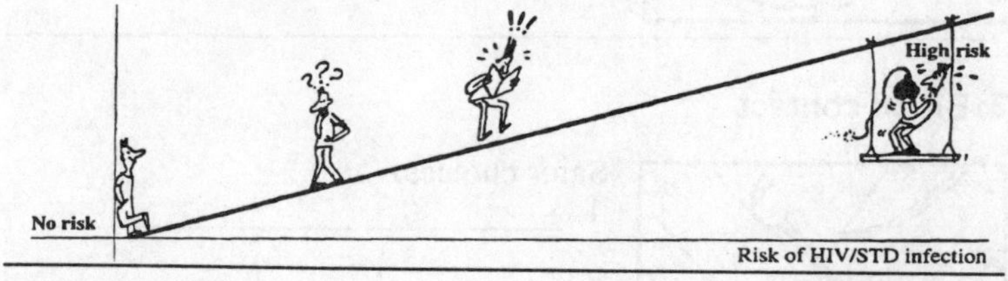

Teacher asks

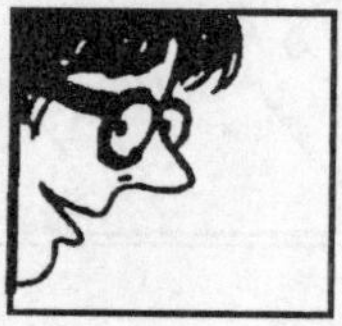

At what other times in your life would it be important to think about your personal risk of getting HIV/STD?

1.10. PROTECT YOURSELF AGAINST AIDS

Why?

We can protect ourselves from STD/HIV and AIDS. We can only do this by making safer choices in how we act. Only this will reduce the risk of coming in contact with the HIV virus.

How?

For each of the three ways of spreading HIV, write safer choices that would protect you from getting HIV.

1. Sexual intercourse

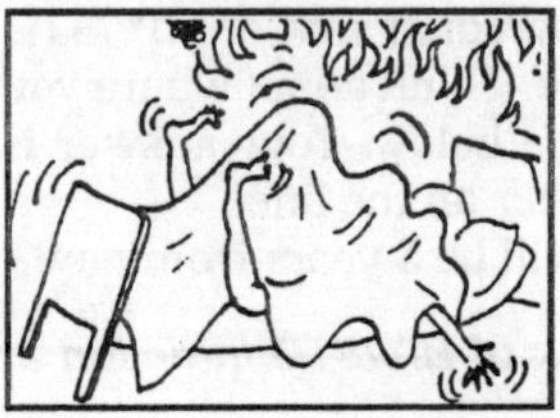

Safer choices:

1. ______________________
2. ______________________
3. ______________________

2. Unsterilized shared needles and syringes

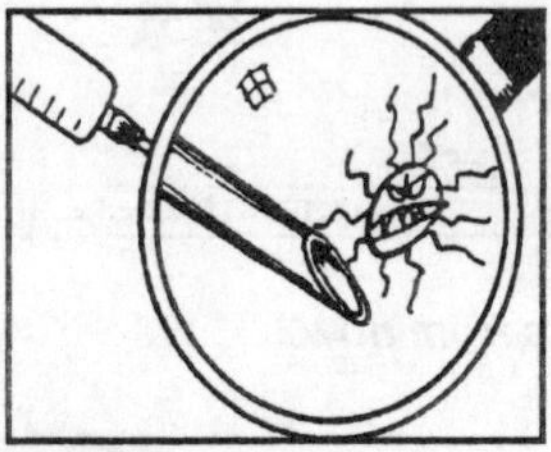

Safer choices:

1. ______________________
2. ______________________
3. ______________________

3. Blood contact

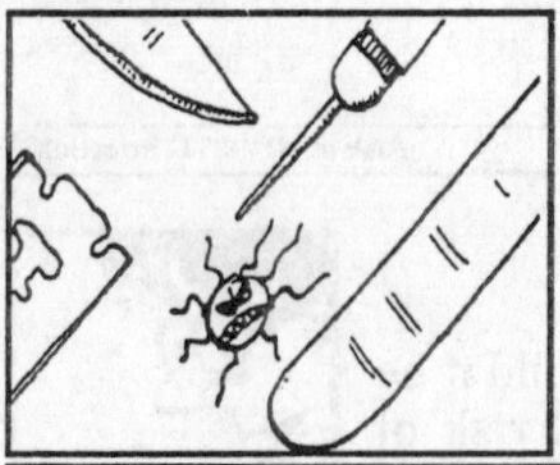

Safer choices:

1. ______________________
2. ______________________
3. ______________________

1.11. DEAR DOCTOR SUE

Why?

It is important for you to learn how to protect yourself from HIV. Doctors and other health workers are a good source of information about protection from HIV/STD.

How?

1. Pretend you are a doctor and must answer each of the letters below.
2. Use the information from the "Doctor's bag" to help you answer the letters.

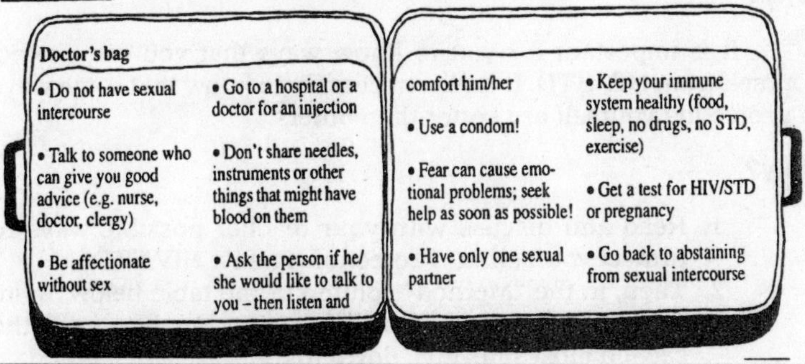

Dear Dr. Sue
I am 14 years old and I have a problem and I don't know who else to turn to. I have been going with a boy for 6 months. Now he tells me we are ready for sex. I told him that I wasn't but now he says I don't love him. He said he will find another girl if we don't have sex. I do love him and I don't want to lose him. He says everyone's doing it.

I'm confused, Norah

Dar Norah,

____

____

____

____

____

____

Dr. Sue

Dear Dr Sue
I am writing to you because I'm worried about my brother. Abrine has left home and is sleeping in the streets with other kids. He doesn 't get much sleep or food and he smokes when he can get cigarettes. He and three friends cut their hands with a knife and touched blood to show they were brothers. He thinks he might have an STD and might need treatment.

Worried, John

Dar John,

____

____

____

____

____

____

Dr. Sue

Dear Dr. Sue,
I hope you can help me. I am a girl 16 years old who has had sex with three different boys and I didn't use any protection. Today we learned at school about AIDS/STD and pregnancy. I think I might be pregnant and now I am very worried about having AIDS or an STD. What can I do ?

Desperate, Allana

Dar Allana,

____
____
____
____
____
____

Dr. Sue

1.12. WHICH IS SAFER?

Why?

It is important for you to know ways that you can protect yourself from HIV/STD. It is also necessary to know that some ways of protecting yourself are better than others.

How?

1. Read and discuss with your teacher possible ways to protect yourself in "Protection against HIV/STD".
2. Then, in the "Method" column of the table below, write the method that is most safe at the top. Then put the second most safe, etc., down to the least safe method.
3. In the "Problem" column, list any problems with the method that might cause a person to get HIV.

Protection against HIV/STD

Reduce the number of sexual partners	Know the other person's sexual history	Show affection without having sexual (petting, kissing, touching)	Have only one sexual partner	Abstain from sexual intercourse	Use a condom every time you have sex	Get tested for HIV

SAFEST

Method	Problem(s)
Least Safe	

1.13. WHAT HAPPENS WITH HIV INFECTION?

This diagram shows the different stages of HIV/AIDS (the timing of stages may vary from individual to individual).

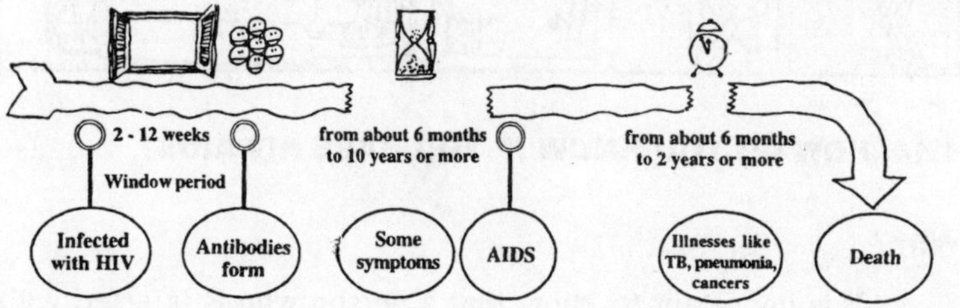

How the person looks

Healthy

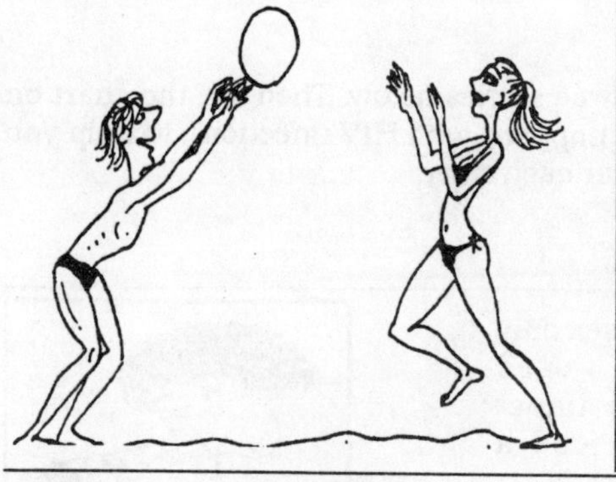

Sick

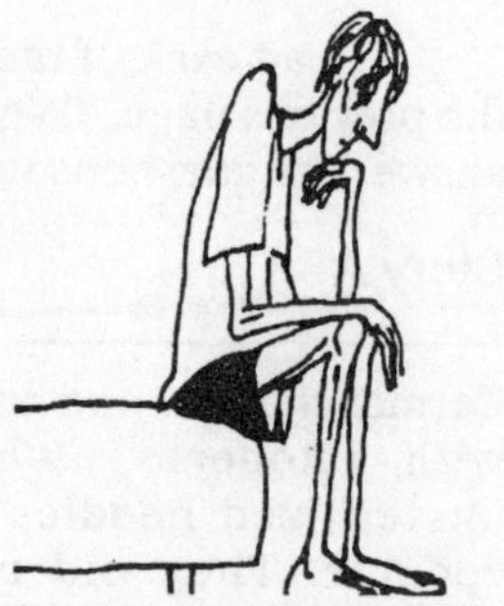

How the person feels

- Most feel very healthy
- Eat normally, can exercise and work
- No or only minor signs and symptoms
- May still be unaware they have HIV
- Can still fight germs
- Some may develop enlarged glands
- May cough and sweat a lot

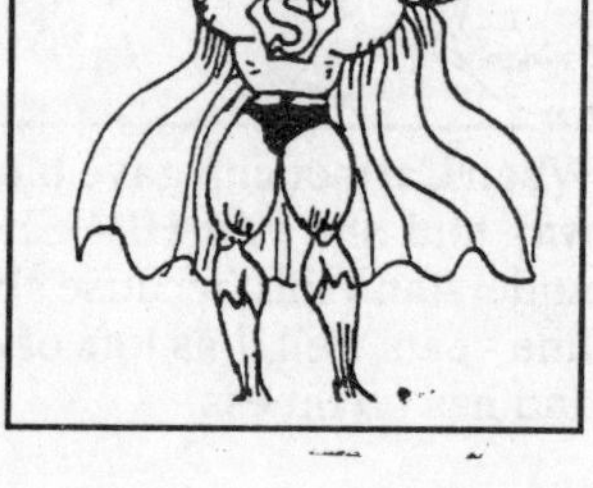

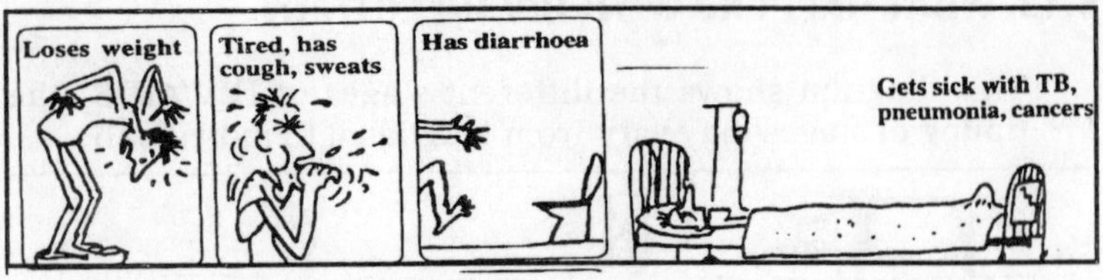
Loses weight
Tired, has cough, sweats
Has diarrhoea
Gets sick with TB, pneumonia, cancers

1.14. HOW DO YOU KNOW IF YOU HAVE HIV/AIDS?

Why?

It is important to know that a person who is infected with HIV:

- May have no signs or symptoms.
- May not have any serious illness for a long time.
- Can infect others during this time.
- Gradually gets sicker and sicker and eventually dies.

How?

Read each of the three stories below. Then use the chart on the previous page, "What happens with HIV infection", to help you answer the questions under each story.

Story A

Carmencita is 17 and had sex only with Roberto who used unsterilized needles to inject cocaine. They did not use a condom.

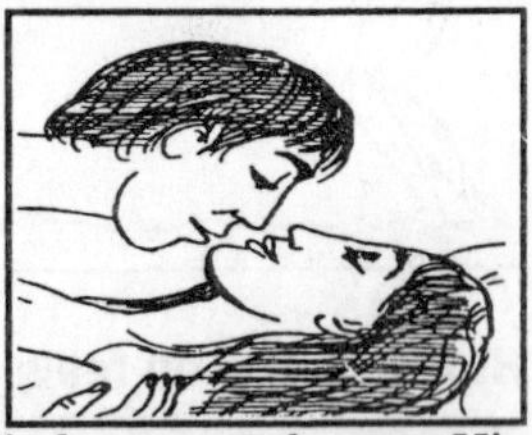

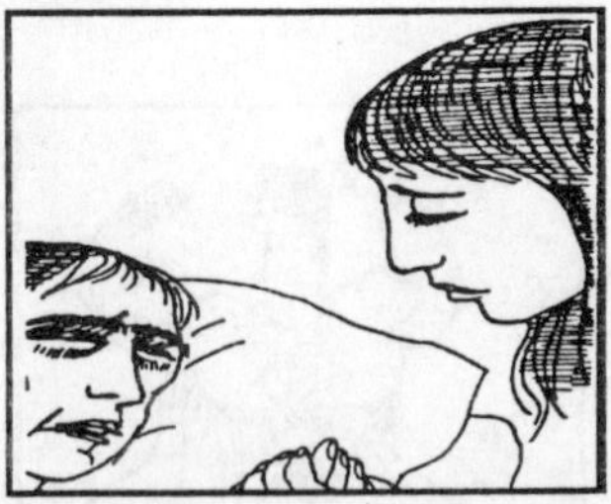

Roberto died two months ago. His last words were, "I hope you don't get AIDS, Carmencita".

When Carmencita gave blood she was told she had HIV. She can't understand this because she feels fine - eats well, has lots of energy and has no illness.

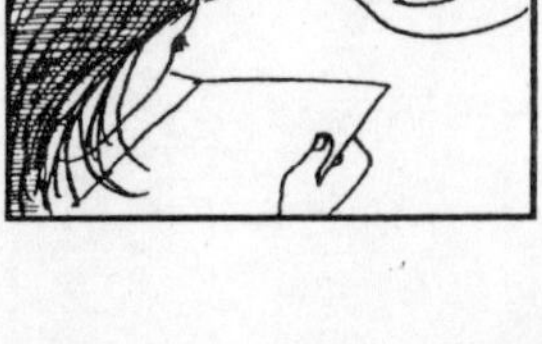

1. How did Roberto become infected? ____________________

____

____

2. How did Carmencita become infected? ____________________

____

3 Why does Carmencita have no symptoms? ____________________

____

4. How long might it be before she gets AIDS? ____________________

____

5. What should Carmencita do now? ____________________

____

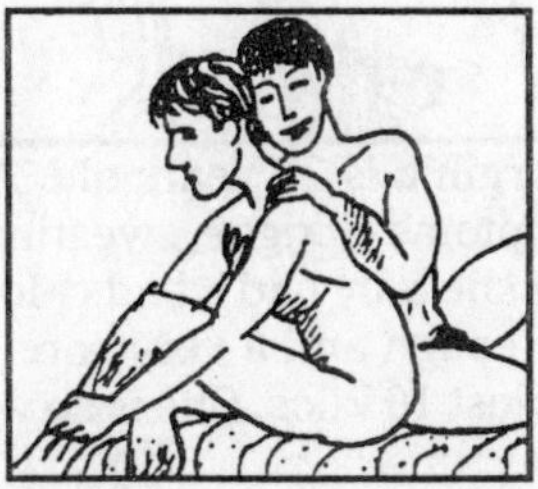

Story B

Jose is 19 years old. He has been having sex with a number of partners without using condoms.

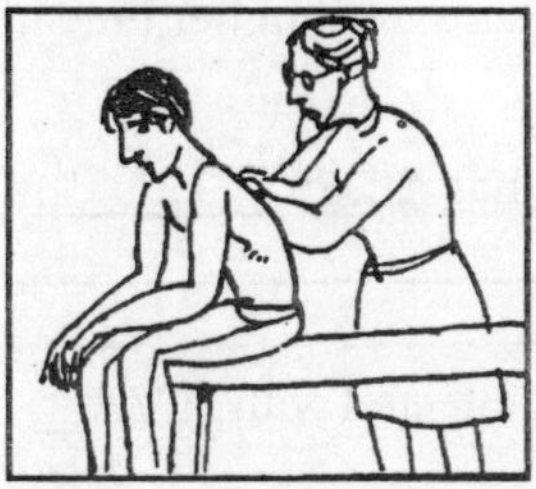

Jose's mother took him to the doctor because he was short of breath, suffered from headaches, and was losing weight even though he was eating normally.

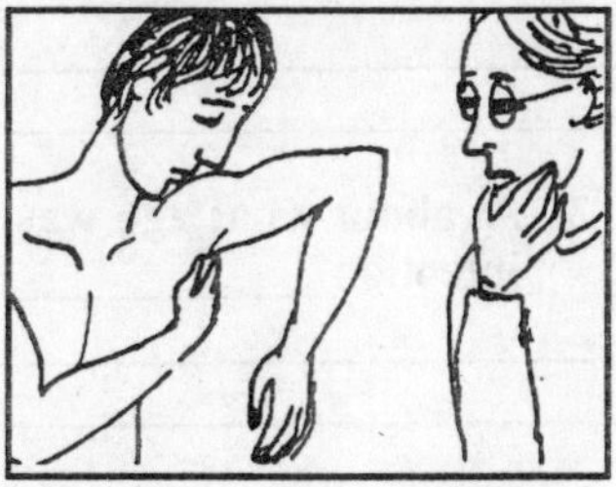

The worst part was waking at night drenched in sweat. He also had chills from a fever and swollen glands under his arms.

1. How did Jose become infected? ____________________

____

2. Why does he have these symptoms? ____________________

____

3. Can he spread HIV to others? How? ____________________

4. What is likely to happen next? ______

Story C

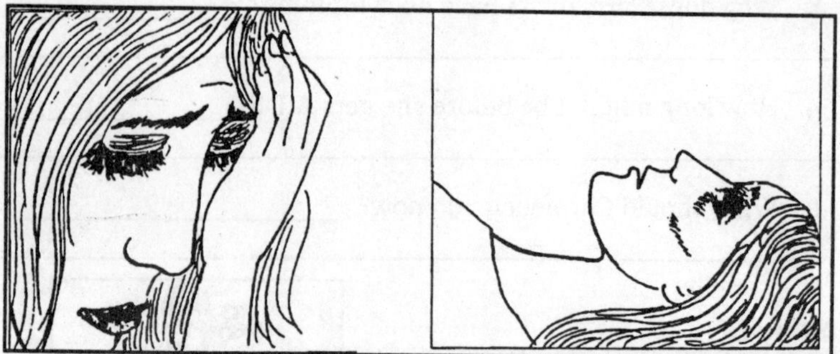

Georginia is 25 years old. About 2 years ago she had a number of symptoms - fatigue, sweating, fever, swollen glands - but she thought that she only had a bad cold or the flu. Now she can't breathe, has a bad cough and a very sore throat. She has stomach problems and has lost 10 kilos. She is so weak that she spends most of her time in bed.

1. Why would you suspect that Georginia has AIDS? ______
2. What should she do to find out if she is infected with HIV? ______
3. At about what age was it possible that Georginia got the HIV infection? ______
4. If she was infected at that age, how long has she been infectious (able to spread HIV)? ______
5. What symptoms does Georginia have? ______

6. What is likely to happen next?

____

____

____

1.15. TESTING FOR HIV

Why?

Some young people may need to know about testing for HIV/AIDS.

How?

Your teacher will help you understand the information below and answer any questions you may wish to ask.

Marie is anxious that she may have HIV from having sex with three partners. She thinks one of her partners might have HIV. She finally got up enough nerve to go to the health centre in her community. She tells the doctor about her situation and asks these questions.

Dr. Matago has worked with people living with AIDS for 7 years. He helps with testing and talks to people who have been tested. He answers Marie's questions in a kind, understanding way.

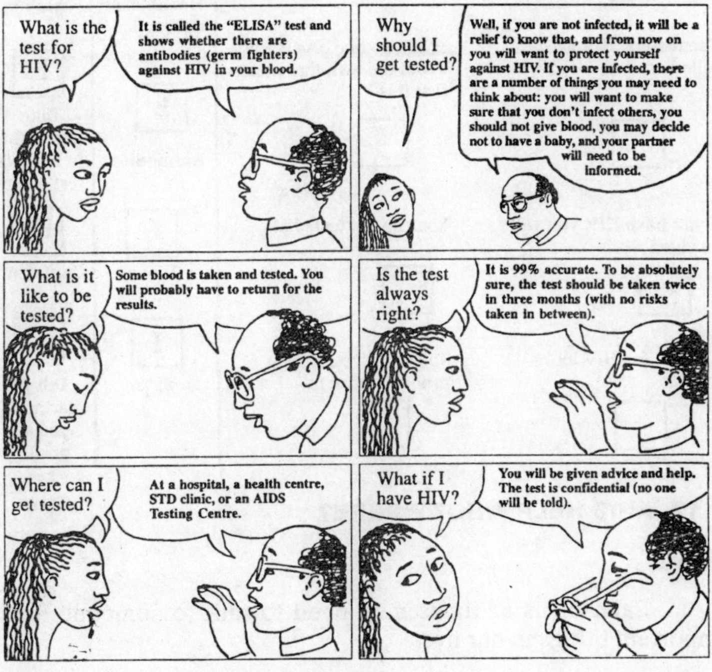

1.16. TEST: WHAT YOU KNOW ...ABOUT TESTING}

Why?

It's important to remember information about HIV/ AIDS and STD. This activity will help you review the information on testing for HIV.

How?

Read the statements in column "A" and try to find the words from column "B" to match the statement.

Column A		Column B	
The number of times you need to be tested in three months is	The test is accurate to	**A** Advice and help	**B** Come back later
It is important to take the test so that you can	It is also important to take the test so that you will	**C** Health centre orhospital	**D** ELISA
The test for HIV is called	When no one else is told about the test, that means that it is	**E** Antibodies	**F** Take precautions to not infect test positive
If you have HIV, you will be given	You can get tested at	**G** Twice	**H** Confidential
The test for HIV looks for......	To get the result syou probably have to	**I** 99%	**J** Tell your partner(s)if you test positive

1.17. AIDS HELP WHO? WHERE?

Why?

Each of us at times may need to talk to someone about important things in our lives.

How?

For each of the situations below, write who you would go to for support and where you would find that help in your community.

1. You have a close friend who is afraid that he/she might have the AIDS virus, HIV.

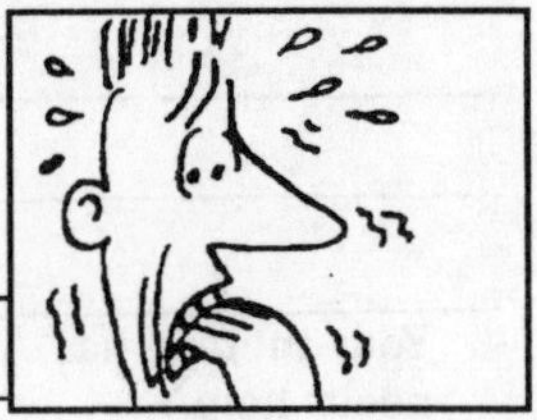

Help from:

____

____

Where or how?

____

____

____

2. After learning about HIV/AIDS in school, you are afraid that you might be infected.

Help from:

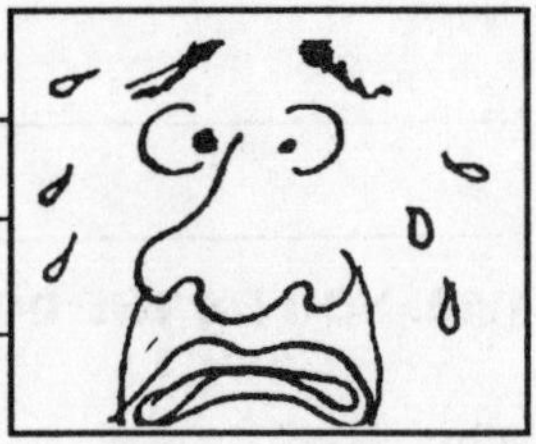

____

____

____

Where or how?

____

____

____

3. You are not feeling well. You have been feeling tired, have swollen glands and sweat a lot at night.

Help from:

____

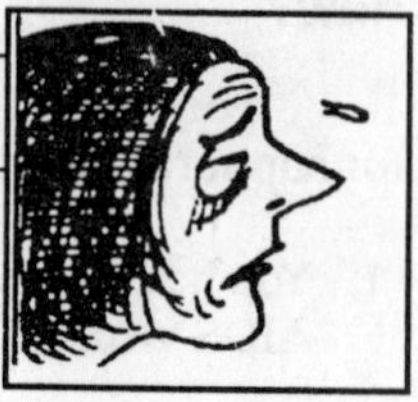

Where or how?

4. Your mother has AIDS, lives alone with you and desperately needs help.

Help from:

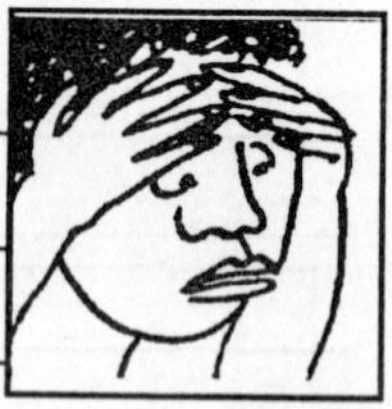

Where or how?

1.18. YOU BE THE DOCTOR

Why

HIV can also be spread through needles used for injecting drugs. It is important know how to protect yourself from getting HIV in this way.

How?

For each of the situation below provide the person with advice from the "Doctor's bag". Use different advice for each case.

Doctor's bag

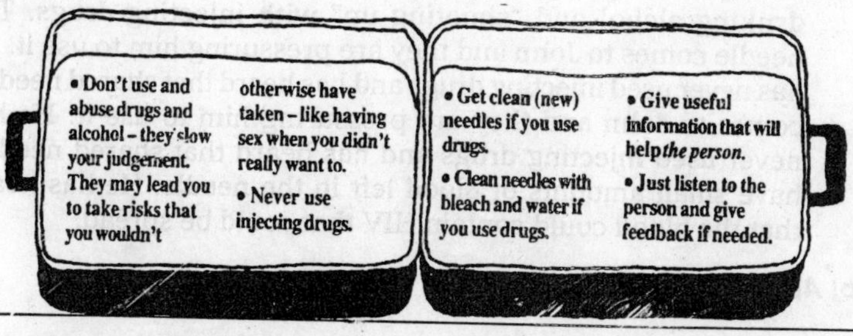

1. Aloha is 16 and was invited to a marriage celebration. There was free alcohol. She had never had much alcohol before but it was hot so she had four of five drinks. She met a young man at the party and he seduced her into having sex. Afterwards, she felt guilty and ashamed that she had been used.

a) Advice

____

____

b) Why?

____

____

2. Jahoa is 17 and lives in the streets since he ran away from home. He has been using injecting drugs (cocaine) for a short time but has never shared needles with others. Today, however, he needs the drugs, but does not have any needles. The health centre is close by and he wonders if they can help him.

b) Advice

____

____

b) Why?

____

____

3. John joins a group of schoolmates in a back street. The are drnking alchol and "shooting up" with injecting drugs. The needle comes to John and they are pressuring him to use it. He has never used injecting drugs and has heard that shared needles comes to John and they are pressuring him to use it. He has never used injecting drugs and has heard that shared needles have small amounts of blood left in the needle. He has heard that the blood could contain HIV that could be spread.

b) Advice

____

____

b) Why?

____

____

4. Jillana has been using injecting needles for three years now and can't stop (she is addicted). She has some drugs but no needle. A friend lends her a needle but she hesitates because she has heard about dirty needles and AIDS.

b) Advice

____

____

b) Why?

____

____

1.19. ARE YOU A RESPONSIBLE PERSON?

Why?

This short test will help you decide if you are a responsible person. Only responsible people can stop HIV and STD.

How?

1. Put a cross in box Yes if you agree, box ? if you are uncertain and box *No* if you disagree.

2. The teacher will discuss the answers with you afterwards so that you can work out your "responsibility score".

Yes Agree	? Uncertain	No Disagree	Statements
☐	☐	☐	1. I keep myself healthy (e.g. do not use drugs)
☐	☐	☐	2. I know how HIV/STD are spread and how to protect myself
☐	☐	☐	3. I would not have sex at this time in my life
☐	☐	☐	4. I would never share needles for drug use
☐	☐	☐	5. When I decide to have sex, I will use a condom
☐	☐	☐	6. When I have sex, I will only have one partner
☐	☐	☐	7. I would tell my partners if I had HIV or STD
☐	☐	☐	8. I would not use unsterilized instruments to pierce my ears, tattoo or shave, etc.
☐	☐	☐	9. I would think hard before having a baby if I or my partner had HIV
☐	☐	☐	10. If I thought I had HIV, I would go to a health centre to ask about tests
☐	☐	☐	11. If a schoolmate or neighbour had HIV or AIDS, I would be a friend to him/her
☐	☐	☐	12. I would get help if I thought I had HIV/STD
☐ +	☐ +	☐	= Total score

Responsibility score

33 - 36 points Very responsible
30 - 33 points Responsible
27 - 29 noints .Somewhat resnonsible
24 - 26 points Not very responsible
24 - O points You are taking risks ! Maybe you should think again.

Unit 2

Responsible Behaviour: Delaying Sex

2.1. REASONS TO SAY NO

Delaying sexual intercourse until: more responsible • older • in a sure relationship with one person • married

There are many good reasons for delaying sex until you are older. These are listed in the pictures below.

How?

Pick 4 reasons young people usually have for abstaining from or delaying sexual intercourse, and place a (√) in these boxes.

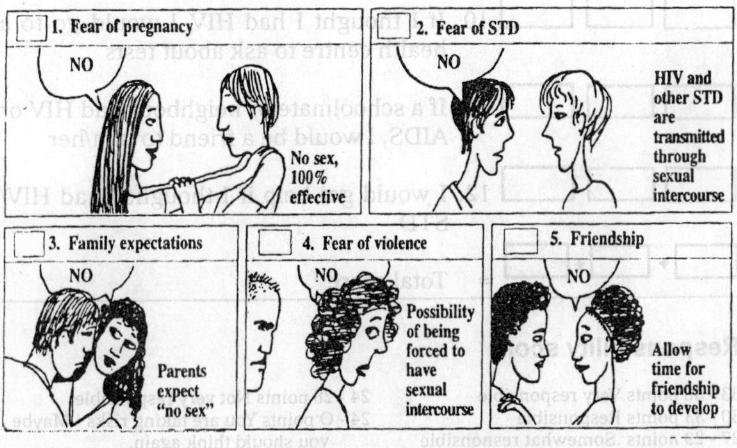
1. Fear of pregnancy
NO
No sex, 100% effective
2. Fear of STD
NO
HIV and other STD are transmitted through sexual intercourse
3. Family expectations
NO
Parents expect "no sex"
4. Fear of violence
NO
Possibility of being forced to have sexual intercourse
5. Friendship
NO
Allow time for friendship to develop

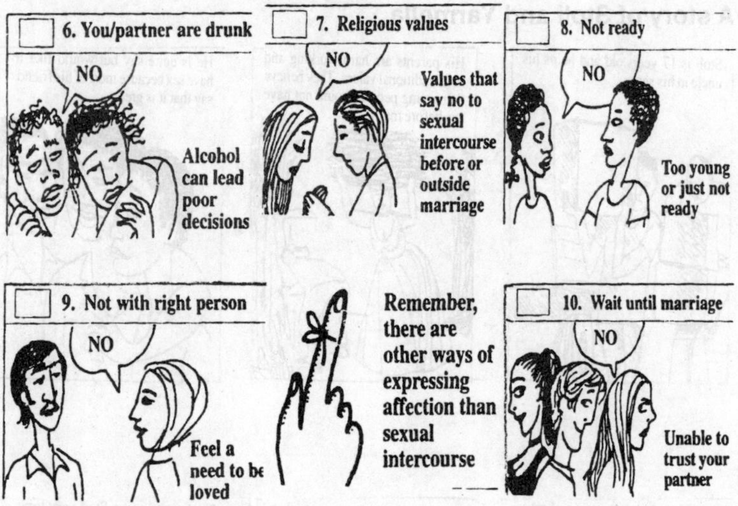
6. You/partner are drunk
NO
Alcohol can lead poor decisions
7. Religious values
NO
Values that say no to sexual intercourse before or outside marriage
8. Not ready
NO
Too young or just not ready
9. Not with right person
NO
Feel a need to be loved
Remember, there are other ways of expressing affection than sexual intercourse
10. Wait until marriage
NO
Unable to trust your partner

2.2. TO DELAY OR NOT TO DELAY (a)

Why?

Decisions about sex are often made in a hurry and sometimes under the influence of alcohol. Decisions about sex should be well thought out. A decision made when calm and not pressured is more likely to result in behaviours that avoid pregnancy and/or HIV/ STD.

How?

1. Read the story of Stoli and Yarmella. From the list of reasons part 1 (next page) for saying "yes" to sex, check those that mig be used by Stoli and Yarmella and then evaluate each reason poor (O) or good (1). Discuss your choice with the rest of the clas
2. From the list of reasons for saying "no" in part 2 (next pagl choose three that might be important for Stoli and three for Yarmell Mark (Y) for Yarmela's reasons to say "no" and (S) for Stoli's.
3. Answer the questions at the end of the activity.

A story of Stoli and Yarmella

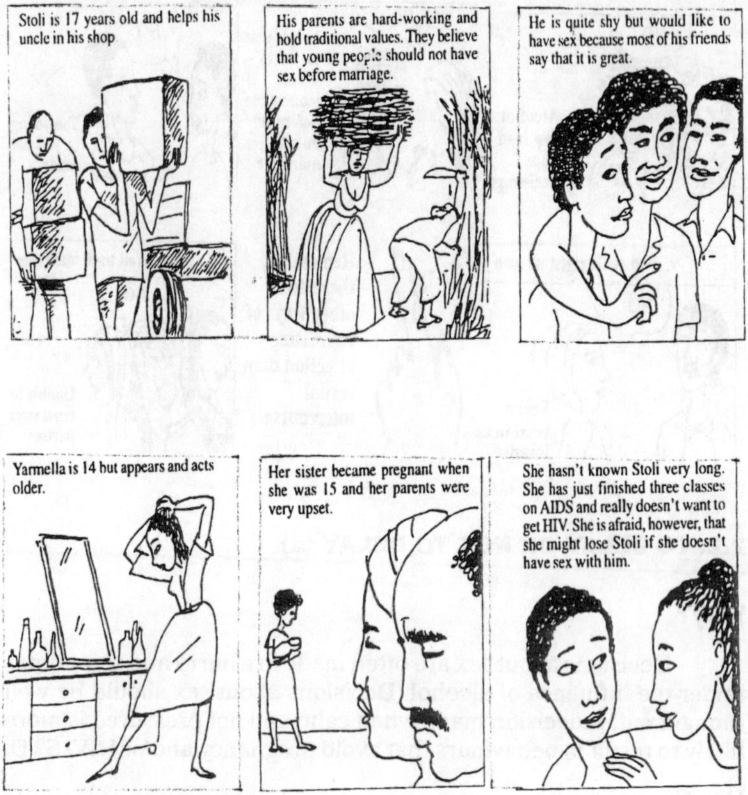

TO DELAY OR NOT TO DELAY (b)

(0=poor reason; 1= good reason)

1 Reasons for saying YES

☐ 1. To prove their love to each other

☐ 2. Fear that the relationship will break up

☐ 3. Curiosity about sex

☐ 4. Belief that everyone is having sex

☐ 5. Because it "feels right"

- [ ] 6. To be more popular
- [ ] 7. Because they are not afraid of be coming pregnant or getting an STD
- [ ] 8. Because both are comfortable with the decision
- [ ] 9. Money or presents
- [ ] 10. Fear of being "beaten up"
- [ ] 11. Because the partner convinces them that there will be no problems

2. Reasons for saying No

(Mark Y for Yarmela's reasons and S for Stoli's).

- [ ] 1. Fear of pregnancy
- [ ] 2. Fear of an STD (like HIV)
- [ ] 3. Family expectations (not to have sex)
- [ ] 4. Fear of cancer (of the cervix)
- [ ] 5. Friendship (to allow to grow)
- [ ] 6. There are other forms of affection
- [ ] 7. Religious values (don't approve of sex)
- [ ] 8. Not ready (perhaps too young)
- [ ] 9. Not with the right person
- [ ] 10. Wait until marriage

Teacher asks

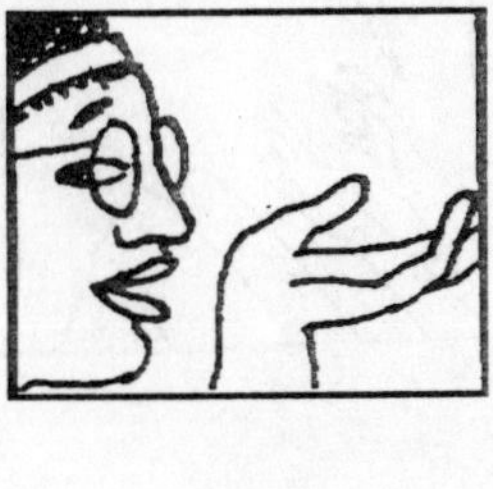

1. How many of your reasons in part 1 were good (1)? How many were poor (O)? How did the rest of the class feel about the reasons for saying "yes"?

2. Did the reasons for Stoli and Yarmella differ in part 2? If yes, why?
3. In part 2 what do you think the one most important reason to delay sex would be for Stoli and for Yarmella?
4. What would be two reasons for returning to abstinence if you were already having sex?

2.3. "LINES" AND MORE 'LINES'

Why?

For every reason to say "no", someone has found a way to persuade you to say "yes". In this activity you learn various ways of replying to these "lines".

How?

1. Read each of the lines to persuade you to say "yes".
2. Using the "Possible responses to Lines and may lines", select the best reply and write the letter in the answer "bubble".

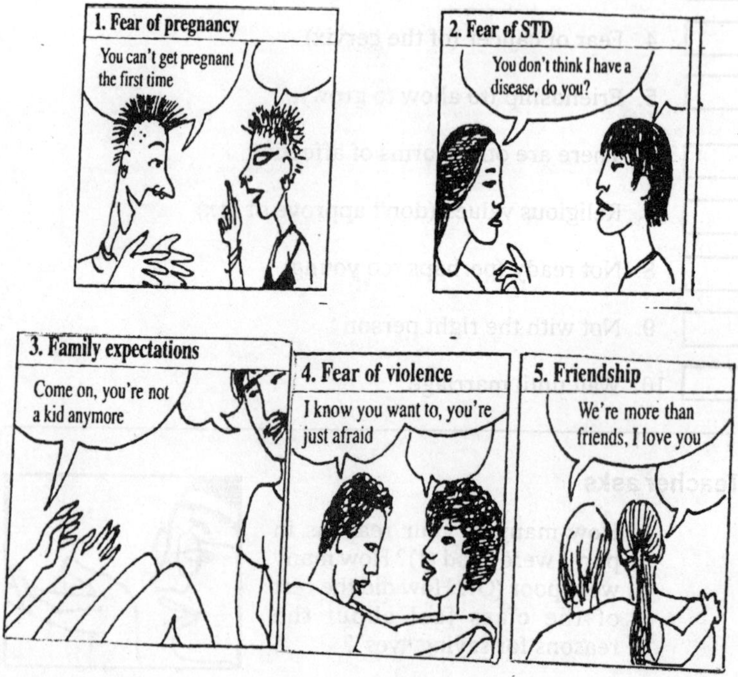

1. Fear of pregnancy
You can't get pregnant the first time
2. Fear of STD
You don't think I have a disease, do you?
3. Family expectations
Come on, you're not a kid anymore
4. Fear of violence
I know you want to, you're just afraid
5. Friendship
We're more than friends, I love you

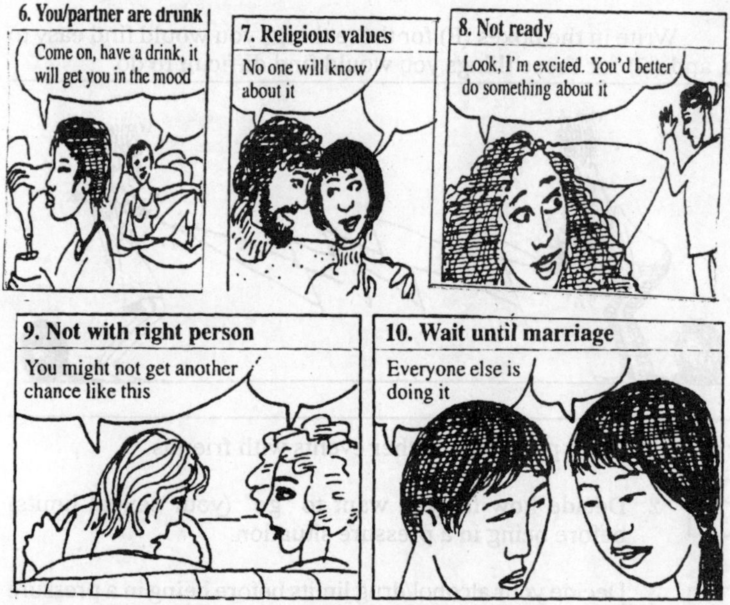
6. You/partner are drunk
Come on, have a drink, it will get you in the mood
7. Religious values
No one will know about it
8. Not ready
Look, I'm excited. You'd better do something about it
9. Not with right person
You might not get another chance like this
10. Wait until marriage
Everyone else is doing it

Possible responses to "Lines and more lines"

A. Once is all it takes.
B. This isn't mjoke. I don't want to get pregnant or get an STD.
C. Maybe we're not ready for sex.
D. I really don't want sex just now.
E. Look, I'm not having sex until I'm older.
F. Maybe we could just hug and kiss.
G. I know that everyone is not having sex.
H. I have no idea, but I'm not taking the risk.
I. I don't feel good when pressured, so I'm leavin,g.
J. No, but *I 'll* know about it.
K. I feel OK about myself without sex.
L. I do too, but I'd like to wait.
M. I don't need a drink, I just don't want sex.
N. I trust *me*, and *me* doesn't want sex.

2.4. GUIDELINES: HELP TO DELAY SEX

Why?

Sometimes it is difficult to say "no" to sex or to delay sex. The guidelines below may help you with these decisions.

How?

Write in the boxes (E) for those things you would find easy to do, and (D) for those things you would find difficult to do.

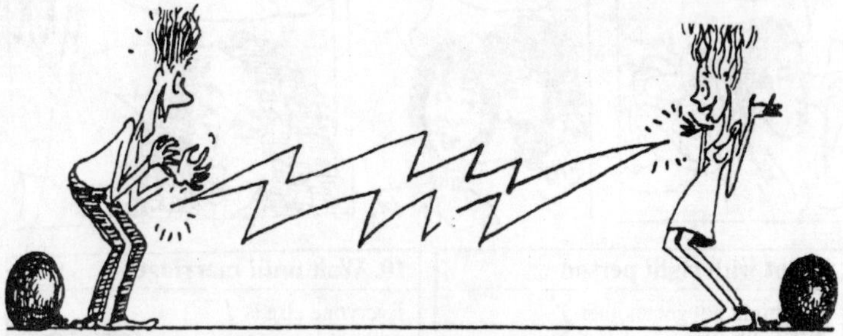

☐ 1. Go to parties and other events with friends.

☐ 2. Decide how far you want to "go" (your sexual limits) before being in a pressure situation.

☐ 3. Decide your alcohol/drug limits before being in a pressure situation.

☐ 4. Avoid falling for romantic words and arguments.

☐ 5. Be clear about your limits - don't give mixed messages, e.g. by acting sexy when you do not want sex.

☐ 6. Pay attention to your feelings; when a situation becomes uncomfortable, leave.

☐ 7. Get involved in activities (e.g. sports, clubs, hobbies).

☐ 8. Avoid "hanging out" with people who might pressure you to have sex.

☐ 9. Be honest from the beginning, by saying you do not want to have sex.

☐ 10. Avoid going out with people you cannot trust.

☐ 11. Avoid secluded places where you could not get help.

☐ 12. Do not accept rides from those you do not know or cannot trust.

☐ 13. Do not accept presents and money from people whom you don't know very well.

☐ 14. Avoid going to someone's room when there is no one else there.

☐ 15. Explore ways of showing affection other than sexual intercourse.

2.5. WHAT TO DO?

Why?

Delaying sexual intercourse is not always easy. But there are things that a person can do which will help delay sex.

How?

1. Read the situations below. From the list under "Help for delaying sex," select three actions that would help each person to delay sex. Write selections in the spaces provided below each situation.

Help for delaying sex

1. Go to parties and other events with friends.
2. Decide how far you want to "go" (your sexual limits) before being in a pressure situation.
3. Decide your alcohol/drug limits before being in a pressure situation.
4. Avoid falling for romantic words and arguments.
5. Be clear about your limits - don't give mixed messages, e.g. by acting sexy when you do not want sex.
6. Pay attention to your feelings; when a situation becomes uncomfortable, leave.
7. Get involved in activities (e.g. sports, clubs, hobbies).
8. Avoid "hanging out" with people who might pressure you to have sex.
9. Be honest from the beginning, by saying you do not want to have sex.
10. Avoid going out with people you cannot trust.
11. Avoid secluded places where you could not get help.
12. Do not accept rides from those you do not know or trust.
13. Do not accept presents and money from people who don't know very well.
14. Avoid going to someone's room when there is no one else there.
15. Explore other ways of showing affection than sexual intercourse.

Situation 1

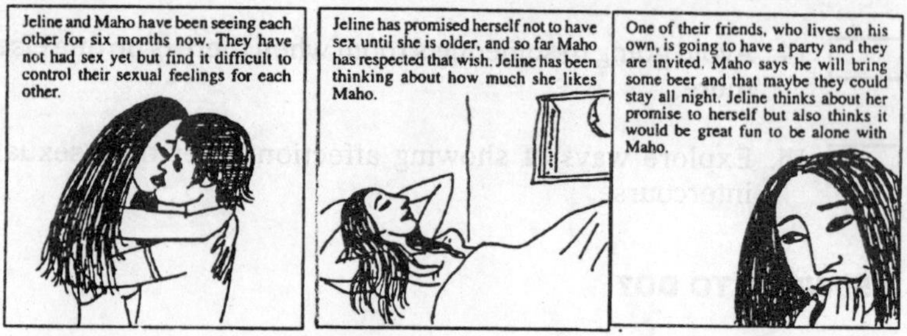
Jeline and Maho have been seeing each other for six months now. They have not had sex yet but find it difficult to control their sexual feelings for each other.
Jeline has promised herself not to have sex until she is older, and so far Maho has respected that wish. Jeline has been thinking about how much she likes Maho.
One of their friends, who lives on his own, is going to have a party and they are invited. Maho says he will bring some beer and that maybe they could stay all night. Jeline thinks about her promise to herself but also thinks it would be great fun to be alone with Maho.

___

Help for Jeline

1. ______
2. ______
3. ______

Situation 2

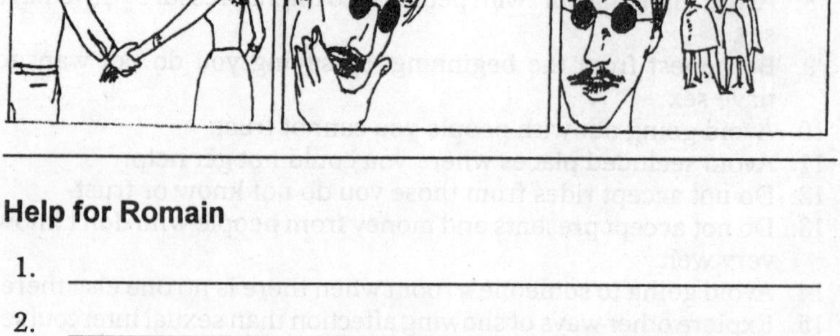

___

Help for Romain

1. ______
2. ______

3. ____________________

Situation 3

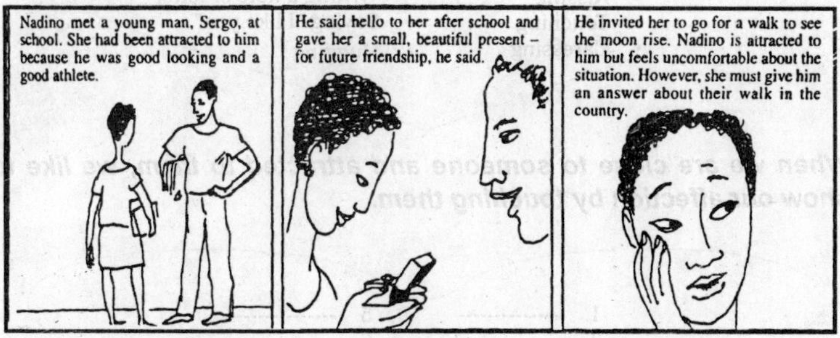
Nadino met a young man, Sergo, at school. She had been attracted to him because he was good looking and a good athlete.
He said hello to her after school and gave her a small, beautiful present – for future friendship, he said.
He invited her to go for a walk to see the moon rise. Nadino is attracted to him but feels uncomfortable about the situation. However, she must give him an answer about their walk in the country.

Help for Nadino

1. ____________________

2. ____________________

3. ____________________

2.6. AFFECTION WITHOUT SEX?

Why?

There are a number of ways of showing affection without having sex. These ways avoid the risk of HIV/STD and unplanned pregnancy.

How?

Students from other schools have come up with a list of ways of showing affection without having sexual intercourse (see the first heart). In pairs or in a small group discuss other ways of showing affection without having sexual intercourse, and write them in the empty lines of the second heart.

- Giving a flower
- Kissing
- Touching
- Caressing
- Holding hands
- Writing a note or letter
- Saying "I like you"
- Hugging

When we are close to someone and attracted to them, we like to show our affection by touching them.

1. --------------
2. --------------
3. --------------
4. --------------
5. --------------
6. --------------
7. --------------
8. --------------

Human beings - babies, small children, young people and adults - all need the comfort of touch; it feels good to be touched by someone we like.

2.7. WHAT'S NEXT?

Why?

Physical affection can be very sexually arousing. The more sexually arousing the activity is, the more likely it will eventually lead to sexual intercourse. If you want to delay sex, it is important for you and your partner to know your limits...

Where should you stop before it leads to sex?

How?

1. Place each of the sexual behaviours from the list of "Physical affection activities" in the appropriate level, from the one that is least physical (1) to the one that is most physical next to sexual intercourse (7).
2. Then answer the questions in "Teacher asks".

Physical affection activities:

Hugging • Touching breasts and/or genitals on top of clothes • Dry kissing • Holding hands • Touching breasts and/or genitals under clothes • Deep (wet) kissing • Body rubbing with no clothes

---

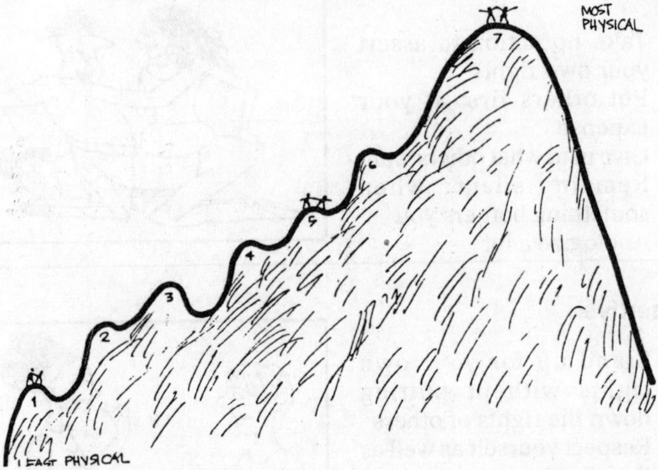

Teacher asks

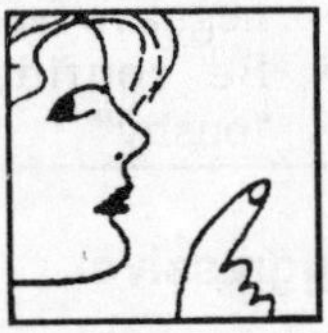

1. Why is it hard to stop as you get closer physically?
2. Would it be easy to go back to a safer activity? Why or why not?
3. Where do you think the limit is?
4. Who should decide where the limit is? When should this limit be decided?

2.8. AM I ASSERWE?

Why?

You are assertive when you stand up for your personal rights without putting down the rights of others. If you can do this you will be able to: 1) Say "no" without feeling guilty; 2) Disagree without becoming angry; 3) Ask for help when you need it. As a result you will feel better about yourself and have more honest friends and relationships.

How?

Your teacher will help you to understand these three types of behaviour.

Passive

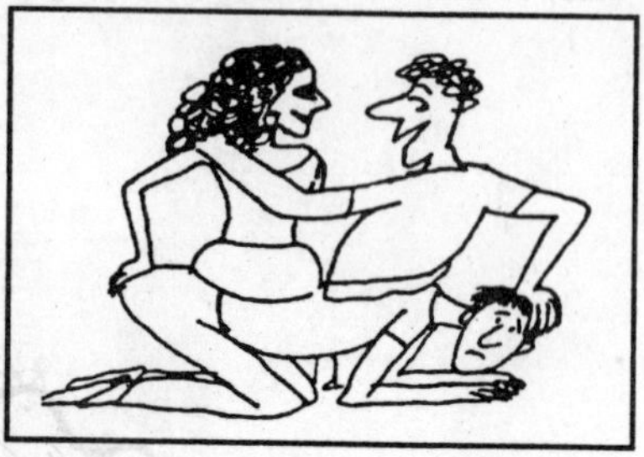

- Take no action to assert your own rights
- Put others first at your expense
- Give in to what others want
- Remain silent when something bothers you
- Apologize a lot

Assertive

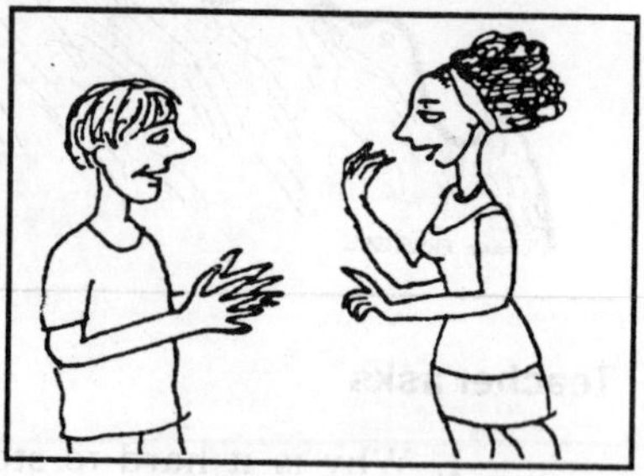

- Stand up for your own rights without putting down the rights of others
- Respect yourself as well as the other person
- Listen and talk
- Express positive and negative feelings
- Be confident, but not "pushy"

Aggressive

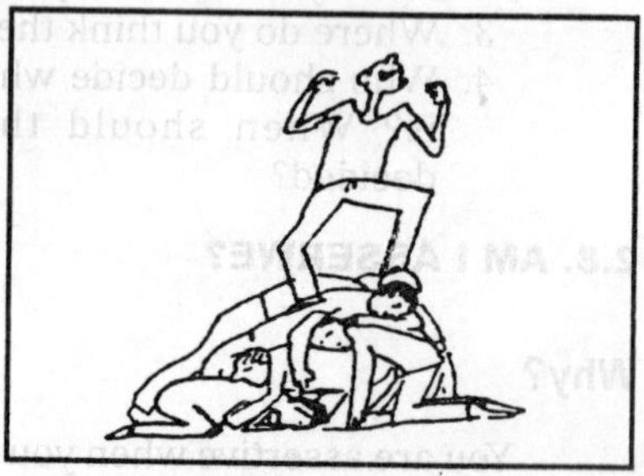

- Stand up for your own rights with no thought about the other person
- Put yourself first at the expense of others
- Overpower others
- Get your own goals, but at the expense of others

2.9. WHO'S ASSERTIVE?

Why?

Since you now know the differences between being passive, aggressive and assertive, it is important to see if you can identify these differences in real-life stories.

How?

1. Read the two stories below.
2. Identify the type of behaviour (passive, aggressive or assertive) of each person in the story.
3. Explain how you identified the type of behaviour by describing: the content of what they said; the way they spoke; their body position.

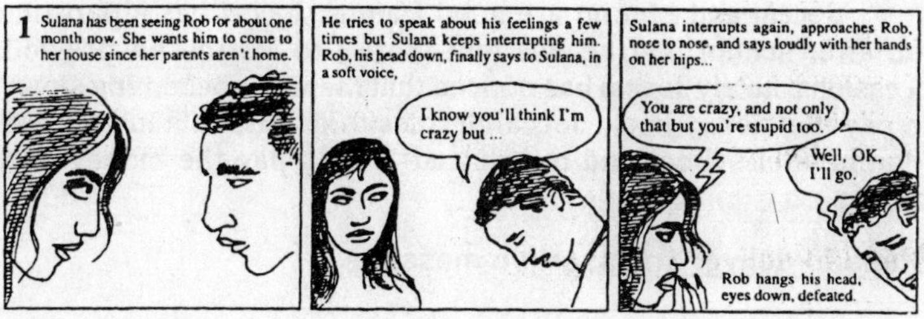
1
Sulana has been seeing Rob for about one month now. She wants him to come to her house since her parents aren't home.
He tries to speak about his feelings a few times but Sulana keeps interrupting him. Rob, his head down, finally says to Sulana, in a soft voice,
I know you'll think I'm crazy but ...
Sulana interrupts again, approaches Rob, nose to nose, and says loudly with her hands on her hips...
You are crazy, and not only that but you're stupid too.
Well, OK, I'll go.
Rob hangs his head, eyes down, defeated.

Rob's behaviour is ____________ Sulana's behaviour is ____________
Why? ____________ Why? ____________
What said? ____________ What said? ____________
How said? ____________ How said? ____________
Body position? ____________ Body position? ____________

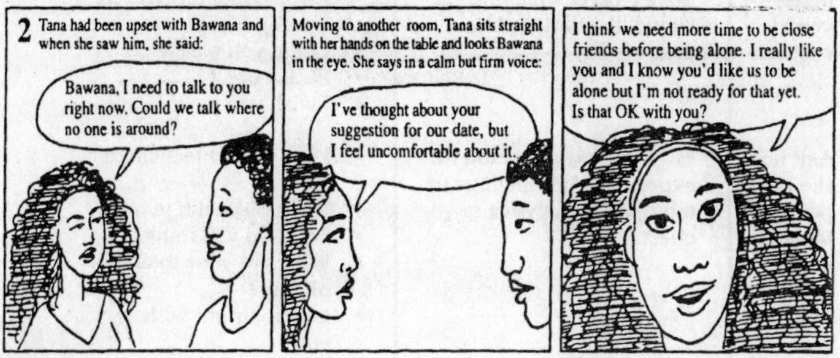
2
Tana had been upset with Bawana and when she saw him, she said:
Bawana, I need to talk to you right now. Could we talk where no one is around?
Moving to another room, Tana sits straight with her hands on the table and looks Bawana in the eye. She says in a calm but firm voice:
I've thought about your suggestion for our date, but I feel uncomfortable about it.
I think we need more time to be close friends before being alone. I really like you and I know you'd like us to be alone but I'm not ready for that yet. Is that OK with you?

Tana's behaviour is ____________
Why? ____________
What said? ____________
How said? ____________
Body position? ____________

2.10. ASSERTIVE MESSAGES

Why?

To be assertive you must first learn the skills. The first time you do this, it will be difffcult. As you practise, it will be easier and feel more natural. Here are the four steps in making an assertive message.

How?

Your teacher will explain the various steps in making an assertive message.

Money problems

Joccai and Mannu are good friends. Joccai has a part-time job after school and he has lent money to Mannu on previous occasions. Lately Joccai has noticed that Mannu is becoming slower to pay the money back. Joccai decides to discuss this matter with Mannu after school and to ask that Mannu pay the money back sooner.

Steps to deliver an assertive message

Steps	Description	Words you might say
1. Explain your feelings and the problem	State how you feel about the behaviour/problem. Describe the behaviour/ problem that violates your rights or disturbs you.	• I feel frustrated when....... • I feel unhappy when....... • I feel. . when .... • I don't like it when.......
2. Make your request	State clearly what you would like to have happen.	• I would like it better if ...... • I would like you to .... • Could you please .... • Please don't .... • I wish you would ....
3. Ask how the other person feels about your request	Invite the other person to express his/her feelings or thoughts about your request.	• How do you feel about that? • Is that OK with you? • What do you think? • What are your thoughts on that? • Is that alright with you?
Answer	The other person indicates his/her feelings or thoughts about the request.	The other person responds.
4. Accept with thanks	If the other person agrees with your request, saying "thanks" is a good way to end the discussion.	• Thanks • Great, I appreciate that • I'm happy that's OK with you • Great

Messages

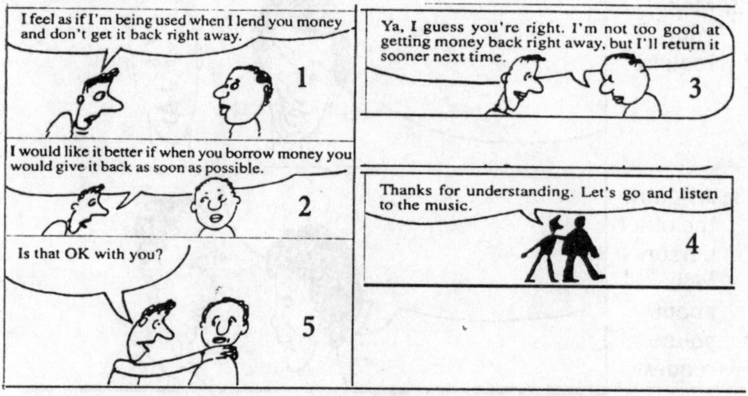
I feel as if I'm being used when I lend you money and don't get it back right away.
1
I would like it better if when you borrow money you would give it back as soon as possible.
2
Ya, I guess you're right. I'm not too good at getting money back right away, but I'll return it sooner next time.
3
Thanks for understanding. Let's go and listen to the music.
4
Is that OK with you?
5

2.11. YOUR ASSERTIVE MESSAGE

Why?

Developing an assertive message as a class will help you understand the steps and prepare you to make your own message in the next activity.

How?

As a class, you will, in this activity, develop an assertive message for the situation described below Your teacher will give instructions.

Dealing with gifts

You are 14 and this is your second date with Adula. He has given you a small gift and he wants to take you dancing. You do not want to have sex with Adula but you think he will want to because of the gift. You decide to tell him that you don't want the gift and you don't want to go to the dance.

Steps to deliver your assertive message

Steps	Your messages
1. Explain your feelings and the problem	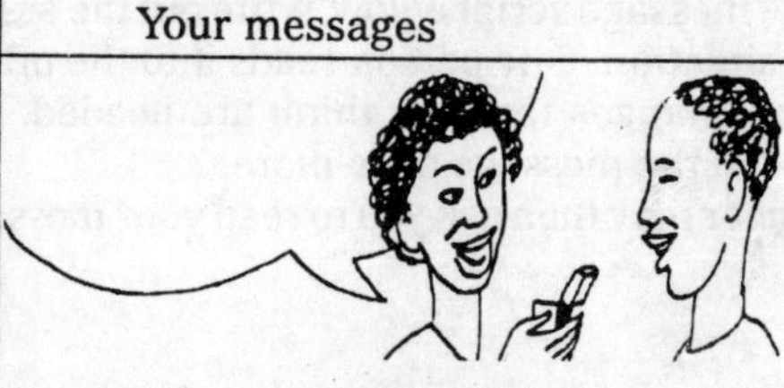

2. Make your request	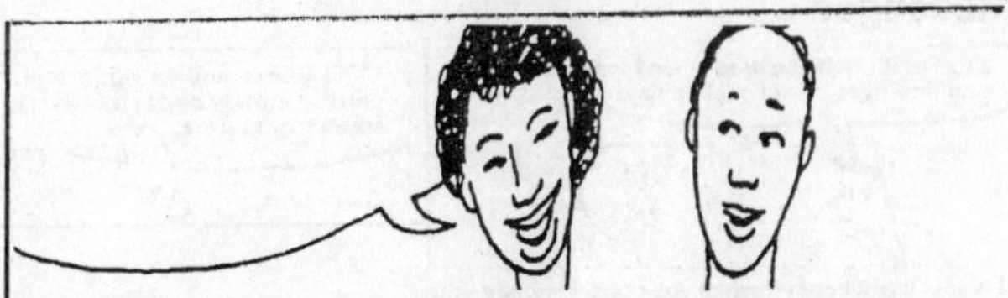
3. Ask how the other person feels about your request	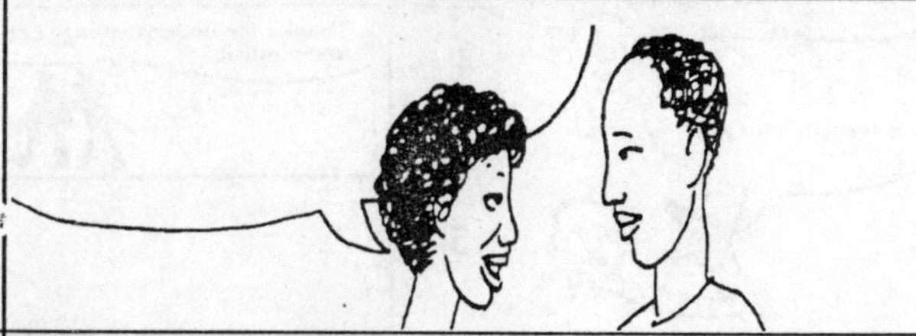
Answer	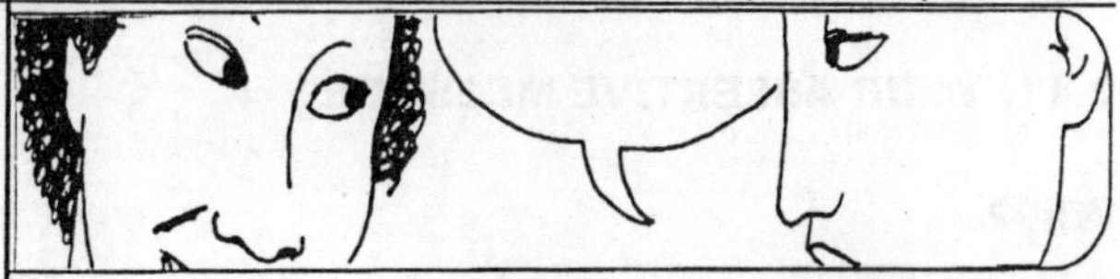
4. Accept with thanks	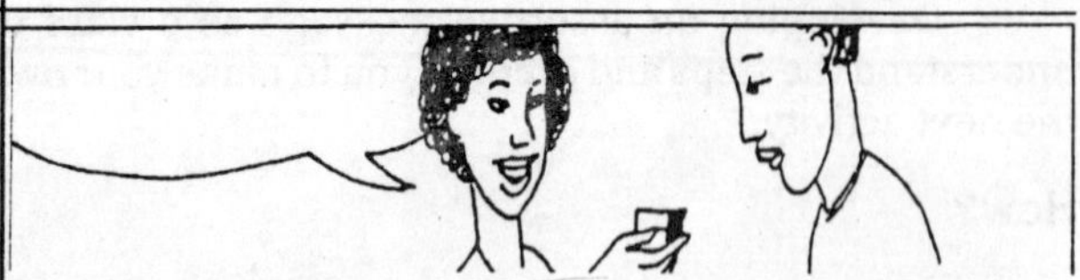

2.12. YOUR ASSERTIVE MESSAGE

Why?

It is now time to try your own assertive message. Remember it may seem awkward at first but it will get better.

How?

1. You and your partner will pick one of the situations from the next page.
2. Using the message script below, write out the assertive message for your situation. One person reads it to the other.
3. Make any changes that you think are needed. Have the other person read the message once more.
4. Your teacher may then ask you to read your message to the class.

Steps to deliver an assertive message

Steps	*Situation 1*	*Situation 2*	*Situation 3*	*Situation 4*
1. Explain your feelings and the problem				
2. Make your request				
3. Ask how the other person feels about your request				
Answer				
4. Accept with thanks				

Sample situations

Situation 1	
You are talking to a number of your friends. Most of them have had sex and are teasing you about the fact that you have not. One of the group hurts you by what they have said. You decide to make an assertive reply.	

Situation 2	
A person of the other sex has asked you to go to a party with him/her. You don't know anyone who is going, which makes you feel a little uncomfortable. As well, you have heard that this person uses drugs and does not have a very good reputation at school. You decide to be assertive and say no to him/her.	

Situation 3

You have decided to get a tattoo or your ears pierced. Your friend has told you that you can get it done at a place out of town. You arrive but it doesn't look very clean. You have heard about HIV/AIDS and unclean needles. You decide to ask the person if the needles are clean and to see the equipment they use for cleaning. When the person can't show you, you decide to say no assertively.	

Situation 4

A friend of your family asks if you want a ride home after school. You don't feel very good about this person and you feel uncomfortable about the situation. You decide to be assertive and refuse the ride.	

2.13. RESPONDING TO PERSUASION

Why?

Other people will not always agree with you when you are assertive. In fact they may interrupt you, get you off the topic or try to persuade you to do something you don't want to do. Therefore, it is important for you to learn how to respond to these situations.

How?

Your teacher will help you to understand how to respond to people who try to get you off the topic or try to persuade you to do something you don't want to do.

Ways people get you off your message or do not accept it

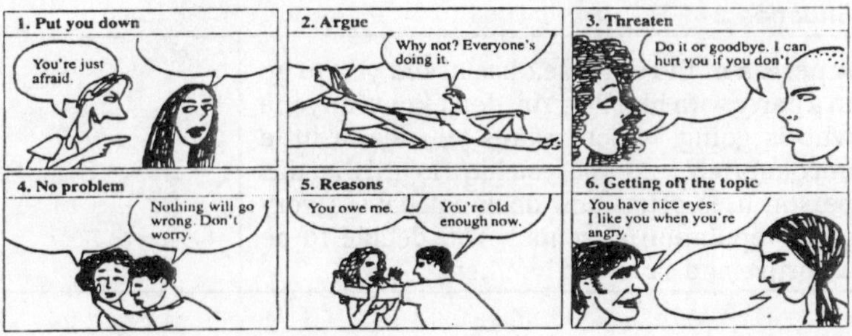
1. Put you down
You're just afraid.
2. Argue
Why not? Everyone's doing it.
3. Threaten
Do it or goodbye. I can hurt you if you don't.
4. No problem
Nothing will go wrong. Don't worry.
5. Reasons
You owe me.
You're old enough now.
6. Getting off the topic
You have nice eyes. I like you when you're angry.

What you say when they...

... try to get you off the topic

In all cases when a person is try ing to get you off your assertive message, get back on topic.

Some ways to do that:

- Please let me finish what I was saying
- Please don't stop me until I'm finished
- That's fine, but please listen to what I have to say
- I know you think ... but let me finish what I was saying

... try to persuade you

If the other person tries to persuade you to do something you do not want to do:

Say no clearly, and if necessary, leave.

Refuse

- No, no, I really mean no
- No thank you
- No, no and I'm leaving

Put off a decision until you can think about it.

Delay

- I' m not ready yet
- Maybe we can talk later
- I'd like to talk to a friend first

Try to make a decision that both people like.

Bargain

- Let's do ... instead
- I won't do that, but maybe we could do ...
- What would make us both happy?

RESPONDING TO PERSUASION

Why?

Learning how to respond to a person who tries to distract you or persuade you to do something that you do not want to do, is an important skill.

How?

Your teacher will explain the steps to take when a person distracts or persuades you.

Situation

Your older brother is supposed to give you a ride home after work.You meet him but he is staggering and slurrinsy his words.You feel he has had too much to drink and it would not be wise to drive with him. He tries to persuade you to go with him. So you refuse, delay or bargain.

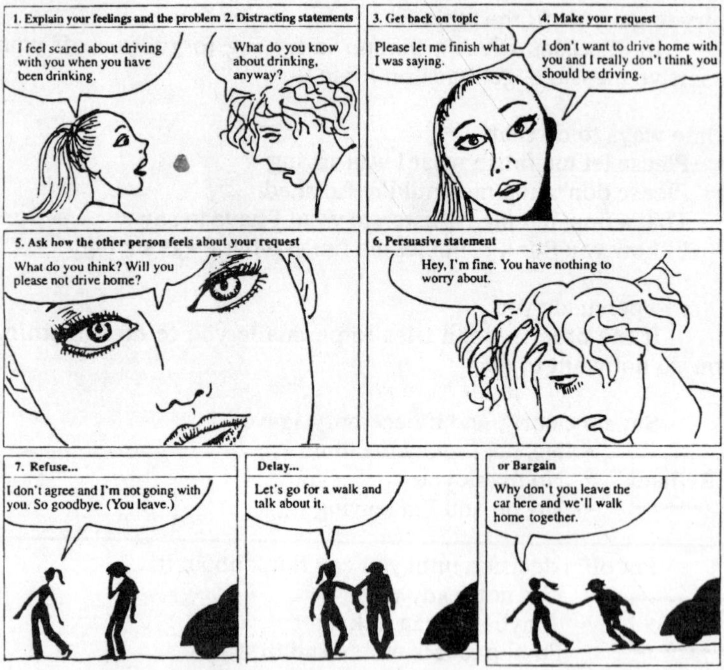
1. Explain your feelings and the problem
I feel scared about driving with you when you have been drinking.
2. Distracting statements
What do you know about drinking, anyway?
3. Get back on topic
Please let me finish what I was saying.
4. Make your request
I don't want to drive home with you and I really don't think you should be driving.
5. Ask how the other person feels about your request
What do you think? Will you please not drive home?
6. Persuasive statement
Hey, I'm fine. You have nothing to worry about.
7. Refuse...
I don't agree and I'm not going with you. So goodbye. (You leave.)
Delay...
Let's go for a walk and talk about it.
or Bargain
Why don't you leave the car here and we'll walk home together.

2.14. RESPONDING TO PERSUASION

Why?

Developing an assertive message as a class will help you understand the steps in responding to distracting or persuading statements.

How?

As a class you will, in this activity, develop an assertive message to use with someone who is trying to get you to do something you don't want to do. Use the situation on the next page. This will help you make your own message in the next activity.

Steps	Words you might say
1. Explain your feelings and the problem	• I feel frustrated when • I feel unhappy when • I feel....... when • It hurts me when ... • I don't like it when ...
2. Distracting statements	Other person tries to get you off topic.
3 Get back on topic	• Please let me finish what I was saying • I'd like you to listen to what I have to say
4. Make your request	• I would like it better if • I would like you to • Could you please • Pleasedon't • I wish you would
5. Ask how the other person feels about your request	• How do you feel about that? • Is that OK with you? • What do you think? • What are your thoughts on that? • Is that all right with you?
6. Persuasive statement	Other person tries to get you to change your mind.
7. Refuse	• No, no, I really mean no • No, no and I' m leaving • No, I'm not going to do that
Delay	• I'm not ready now - maybe later • Maybe we can talk later • I'd like to talk to a friend
Bargain	• Let's do ... instead • How about we try • What would make us both happy?

Situation

You are alone with your boyfriend at his house. It is night and he lives quite a distance from your home on a deserted road. He is usually very gentle but tonight he has been drinking beer. He becomes quite aggressive with his demands for sex. He interrupts you and tries to talk you into having sex. You refuse, delay or bargain.

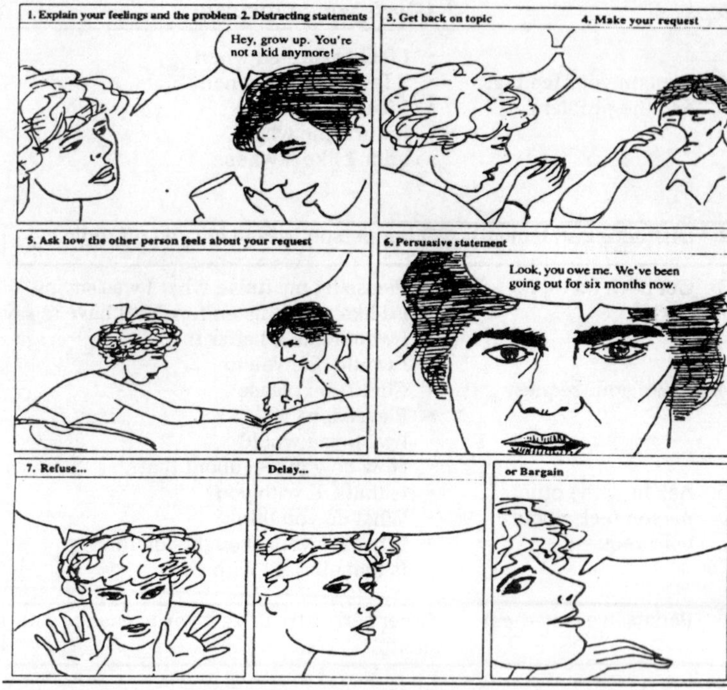
1. Explain your feelings and the problem
2. Distracting statements
Hey, grow up. You're not a kid anymore!
3. Get back on topic
4. Make your request
5. Ask how the other person feels about your request
6. Persuasive statement
Look, you owe me. We've been going out for six months now.
7. Refuse...
Delay...
or Bargain

Question

Should you refuse and leave in this situation? You are far from home and it is dark. What else could you do?

2.15. RESPONDIG TO PERSUASION

Why?

In this activity, you'll try to write an assertive message to someone who interrupts you and tries to get you to do something you don't want to do.

How?

1. With a partner, use the blank spaces to write an assertive message.
2. Select a statement that tries to get you to do something that you don't want to do.
3. Finally, write a "refuse", "delay" or "bargain" statement.

Situation 1

Your friend wants you to skip school and go to the river to drink beer. He tells you a whole group is going. He says, "You are afraid, aren't you". You got caught skipping school last month and don't want to get caught again. You decide to tell him you don't want to go.

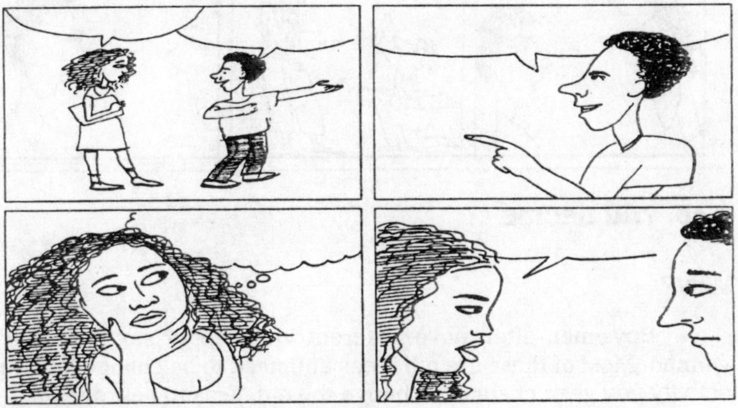

RESPONDING TO PERSUASION

Situation 2

Your parents are at work and you invite a friend of the opposite sex over to study. After doing the homework he/she grabs you and tries to kiss you. You push him/her away but they say, "Come on, you didn't invite me over just to do homework." You take a firm stand so it won't happen again.

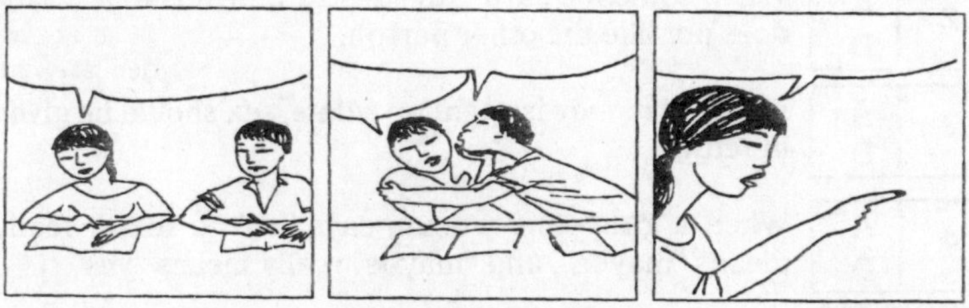

Situation 3

Your boyfriend/girlfriend thinks it is time to have sex. You love him/her but you feel that sex before you are ready is wrong.

Your friend says, "You're just scared. If you really loved me, you'd show it." Although you are afraid it will end the relationship, you decide to tell him/her that you are just not ready.

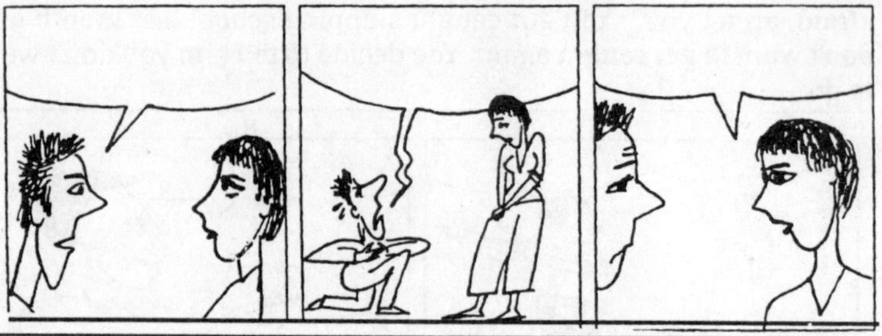

2.16. YOU DECIDE

Why?

Boys/men often have different ideas about sex from girls/ women. Most of these are old ideas and need to be changed. In this activity you get a chance to change the old ideas to new ones.

How?

1. Circle A (agree) if you think the statement is correct or right for you.
2. Circle D (disagree) if you think the statement is incorrect or wrong for you or is not the right way to think.

1	A D	The success of an evening out with a young woman/ young man can be judged by how sexual it was.
2	A D	When someone says "No" to sex, it means that he/she does not like the other person.
3	A D	If a lot of money is spent on a date, sex should be given in return.
4	A D	When a girl/young woman says "no" to sex, it really means "maybe", and "maybe" really means "yes".
5	A D	A real man is one who has had sex with a woman.
6	A D	Someone who dresses in a sexy way wants to have sex.

7	A D	If a girl/boy accepts an invitation to go to somebody's house alone, she/he would be expected to have sex.
8	A D	It is the woman's responsibility to decide how sexual a relationship becomes.

New statement

3. Finally, write a new statement that you think would be better for both boys/men and girls/women.

The success of an evening out should be judged on...

When a person says no to sex, it means...

If a lot of money is spent on a date it does not mean...

No to sex really means...

You are a real man if...

If someone dresses or acts in a sexy way...

If a person wants to go to someone else's house when there is no one else home...

It is...

...responsibility to set sexual limits

2.17. DEALING WITH THREATS AND VIOLENCE

Why

Women need to be aware of situations that may lead to violent sex, and people who may put them in those situations. It is important for you to learn ways of avoiding or dealing with pressures and threats to have sex.

How?

1. Read the story of Maria
2. Discuss the questions under "Teacher asks"

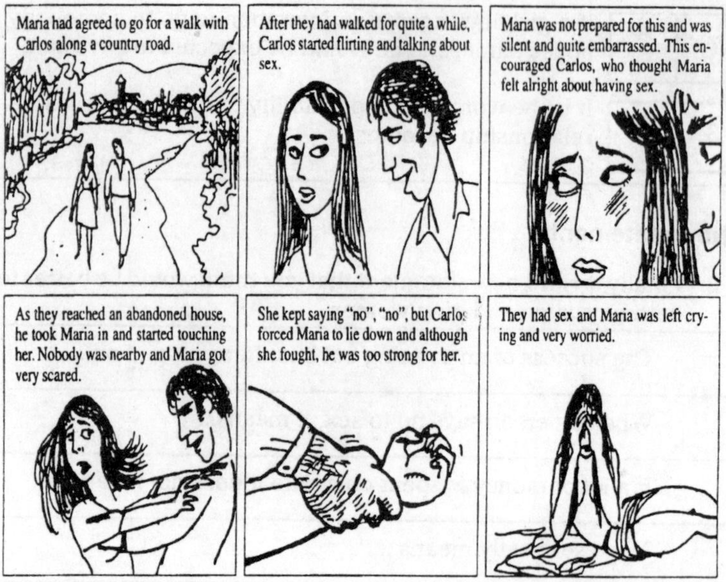

Teacher asks

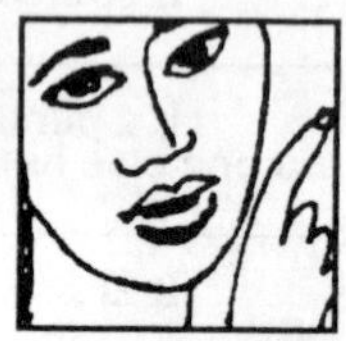

1. Do you think that Maria could have been aware of what was going to happen? What were the clues that could have told her?
2. Maria was silent and embarrassed when Carlos started talking about sex. What could she have done instead of being silent and embarrassed?
3. What should she do now? Keep it a secret? Tell someone she trusts (parents, teachers, religious leader)? Should she talk to Carlos about the matter? What might happen if she doesn't tell anyone about the situation?
4. List things you can do to help prevent violence and threats:
   a) When you're with someone who suggests having sex and you don't want to.
   b) When someone becomes physical and tries to force you to have sex.
5. What do you think about Calors? Are there other men like Carlos? What he have done in this situation? Why did he do what he did?

BEING ASSERTIVE EVERY DAY

Why?

This activity will help you to become assertive in your everyday life. To do this you must decide on one specific situation in which you want to be more assertive. For example, you may want to say "no" to those who pressure you to do things you really don't want to do. To help you in this activity you should set out a plan and then write a short summary of how your plan worked.

How?

1. Complete the action plan below. Select an assertive goal from the list "Possible assertive goals" below, or make up your own.
2. Try your assertive goal for one week and at the end write a short summary of how successful you were at being assertive.

Action	Description	My personal plan
Set a Specifle assertive	Select from the list below or make up your own (e.g. to say "no" when I am pressured to do something).	The assertive goal I have for myself is to:
When will I ractise?	Set a date when you will start and another when you will complete the goal (e.g. Nov. 8 to Nov. 15).	I will start my assertive goal on: and I will finish on:
How will I benefit?	How do you think you will feel about yourself when you have completed your goal (e.g. I will feel better about myself)?	I will probably feel:
How will I reward myself?	When you have finished your week, you should plan to gives yourself something nice (e.g. go to a movie)	I will celebrate my goal by:
Contract with m self	By signing a contract with your-self you are more likely to do what you plan	I will: (put in assertive goal) for one week and will reward myself at the end of the week. Signature: Date:

Possible assertive goals

- To ask someone to do something with me
- To ask people to listen to me when they ignore me
- To tell my friends, brother or sister when they bother me - but in an assertive way
- To be more assertive with my boyfriend or girlfriend
- To say how I feel about things more often
- To express my feelings without putting someone down or criticizing them
- To say no when I don't want to do something
- To say how I feel when people put me down or hurt me

Unit 3

Responsible Behaviour: Protected Sex

3.1. THE CONDOM

Why?

For sexually active people, the condom is the best protection against STD and HIV. Information about condoms is important for positive attitudes and effective use.

How?

Your teacher will discuss these points with you.

Strong • Safe • Sensitive

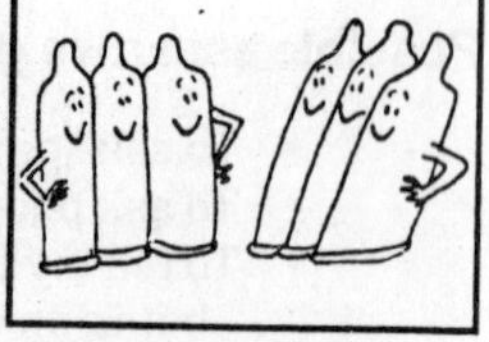

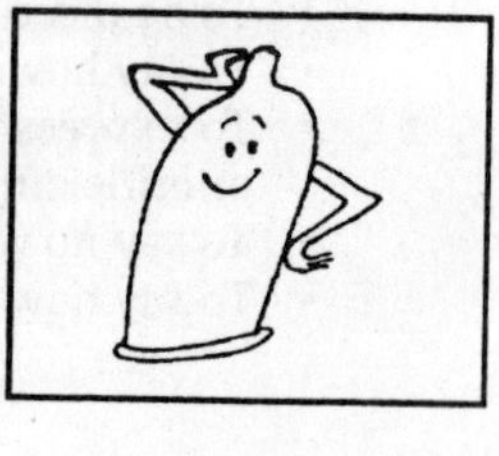

- *Where can you get condoms?* You can buy condoms or sometimes get them free at...
- *Do they come in different sizes?* Usually one size fits all.
- *Can condoms protect you from illness?* Yes; as well as preventing pregnancy, condoms protect you from HIV and other STD.
- *Are condoms safe?* If used properly, they are very safe.
- *Can a condom be used again?* No, a condom should be used once only and then thrown away.

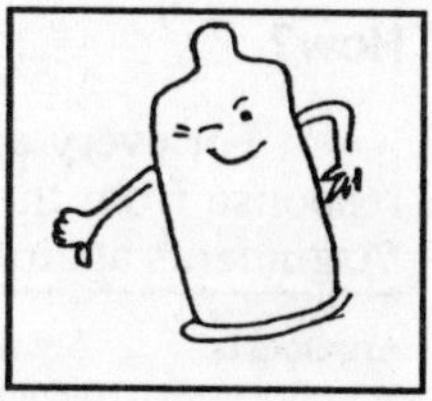

- *Can a condom tear?* Yes, so you must be very careful with your fingernails! And you should be especially careful when opening the package, not to damage the condom inside with your teeth or fingernails.

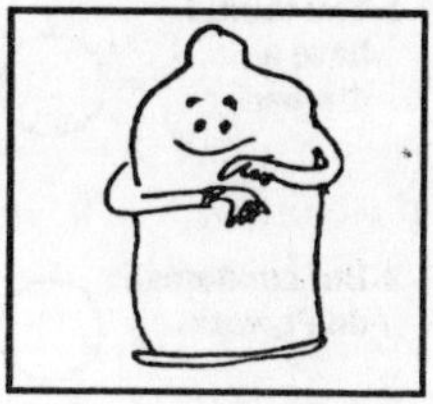

- *How long do condoms keep?* You should never use a condom after the expiry date which is printed on the package. Keep condoms in a cool, dry spot, out of the sunlight.
- *Do condoms reduce sensation?* Nowadays condoms are very thin and at the same time very strong. Stronger does not mean thicker. Condoms these days, hardly reduce sensation.

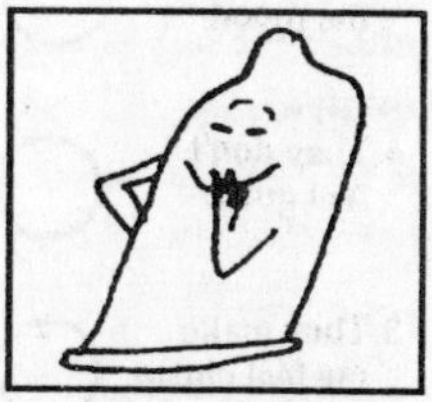

- *Can a condom slip off inside the woman?* Yes, but not if you have put it on properly - read the instructions carefully and practise on your own!
- *Can a woman put a condom on a man?* Yes, women often buy condoms and help put them on the man. The woman and the man should both know how to put condoms on properly.
- *Is there a condom for women?* Yes, a condom has now been invented for women. It fits inside the vagina and prevents any contact with the man's semen.
- *Should you use a lubricant with a condom?* Yes; lubrication helps to avoid tearing. Some condoms are already lubricated. If the condom is not lubricated, use a water-based lubricant - never use vaseline or vegetable oil as these lubricants can damage the condom.

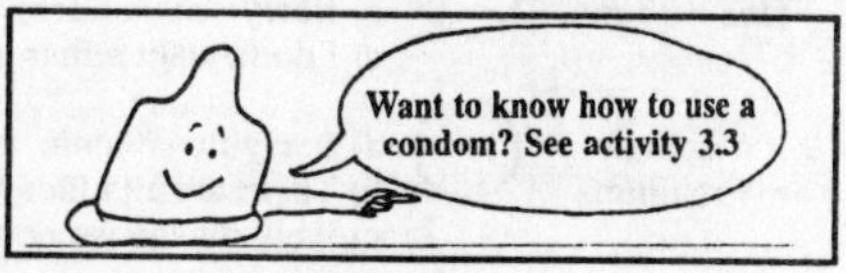
Want to know how to use a condom? See activity 3.3

3.2. ARGUMENTS PEOPLE USE AGAINST USING CONDOMS

Why?

Your partner may not like using condoms. If you want to be safe from STD, HIV and pregnancy it is important to learn how to talk to a person who dislikes using condoms.

How?

For every argument against using condoms choose the best response from the list of three. Place the letter in the circle after "Arguments against".

Arguments	Answer against	Responses
1. You think I have a disease.	◯	a) I don't want either of us to take a chance of getting HIV. b) You know many people infected with HIV have no symptoms at all. c) We probably don't have a disease, but isn't it better to be sure?
2. But condoms don't work.	◯	a) They're OK if we use them the right way. b) Will you try condoms a few times and see? c) They are the best protection available.
3. They spoil the mood.	◯	a) It won't be so bad after we get used to them. b) Hey, condoms may even be fun. c) We can use them together.
4. They don't feel good.	◯	a) It will be OK once we're used to them. b) Will you try condoms a few times and see? c) But it would make me feel more relaxed if I felt safe.
5. They make me feel cheap and dirty.	◯	a) But we know condoms can protect us. b) I know you don't like the idea but condoms are so important now. c) Anyone can get HIV, even people like us.
6. I'm already using pills for birth control.	◯	a) We'll have to use condoms as well, the pill doesn't protect us from infections b) That doesn't help against HIV and STD. c) Too bad - no condom, no sex.
7. I'd be embarrassed to buy one.	◯	a) It won't be so awkward after the first time. b) I'll buy them, so we'll have them next time. c) Embarrassment never killed anyone.
8. I don't have One with me.	◯	a) I'll get one for next time, but today, no sex. b) Sorry - no condom, no sex. c) I don't want either of us to take a chance of getting AIDS.
9. It's against my religion.	◯	a) Sorry-no condom, no sex. b) There are all kinds of things we can do without having sex. c) Well, maybe we're not ready for sex.
10. They cost too much.	◯	a) Sorry, I really care about my health and yours. b) I can help you pay for them. c) Let's not have sex until we can work this out.

3.3. HOW TO USE A CONDOM

Why?

Condoms offer good protection and are unlikely to break, if you know how to use them properly.

How?

Your teacher will give you instructions on how to do this activity.

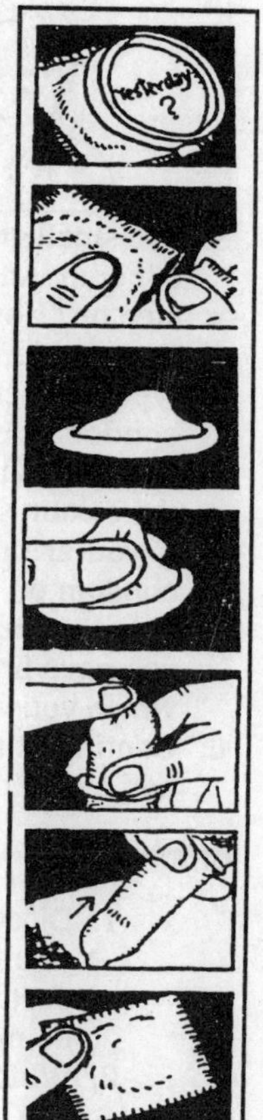

1. Check the expiry date. Store condoms in a cool, dry place.
2. Open package carefully so condom does not tear.
3. Make sure condom is pointing in right direction. Do not unroll condom before putting it on.
4. Squeeze tip of condom.
5. Still holding tip, unroll condom until it covers all of erect penis.
6. After intercourse and ejaculation, hold rim of condom and pull penis out before it gets soft.
7. Dispose of condom in a safe place. Use a new condom next time

3.4. CONDOM PRACTICE

Why?

In this voluntary activity, you can practise putting a condom on a model of a penis (or on a banana or cucumber). This may be an activity that you don't want to do. It is perfectly alright for you to refuse. Whatever your decision, remember that this activity may be helpful some time in the future when you may want to use a condom.

How?

After the activity below, complete the "Teacher asks" section with your small group.

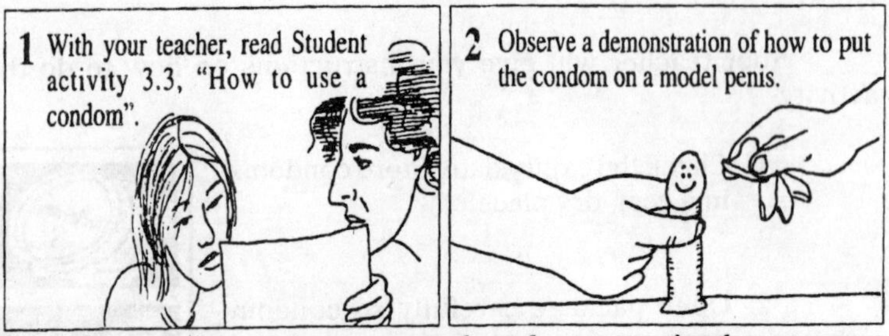
1 With your teacher, read Student activity 3.3, "How to use a condom".
2 Observe a demonstration of how to put the condom on a model penis.

3. In a small group, observe a student demonstrating how to use a condom. Another student should read the instructions for each step on "How to use a condom" (Student activity 3.3).
4. Each student will be given one packaged condom. Observe the type of packaging and the information on the outside of the condom wrapper. Note the expiry date. Open the condom wrapper carefully. Observe how easy it is to open the package; the colour, shape; and lubrication (if any).
5. If you are comfortable with the activity, practise putting the condom on the model. Other group members will help you by either reading each step for you or by judging how you did after you have finished putting the condom on (you should tell them which you would like before you start).
6. Continue these instructions until everyone in your group has had a chance to practise putting the condom on the model.

Teacher asks

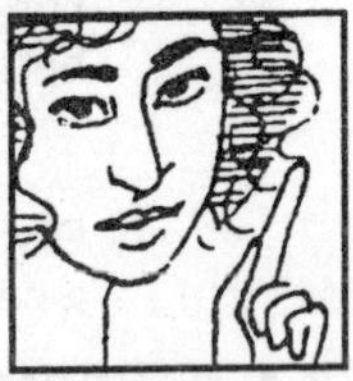

1. Discuss problems that might occur if you were to use a condom with a partner in a real life situation (e.g. not being able to see in the dark);
2. Which was the most difficult part for you? How could you make it easier?

3.5. NO TO UNPROTECTED SEX

Why?

Being assertive when your partner does not want to use a condom is very important. The bottom line is "no sex without a condom".

How?

This situation will show you how to deal with a person who does not want to use a condom. This is done using the assertive skills you learned earlier.

"We're both clean... We don't need to use a condom!"

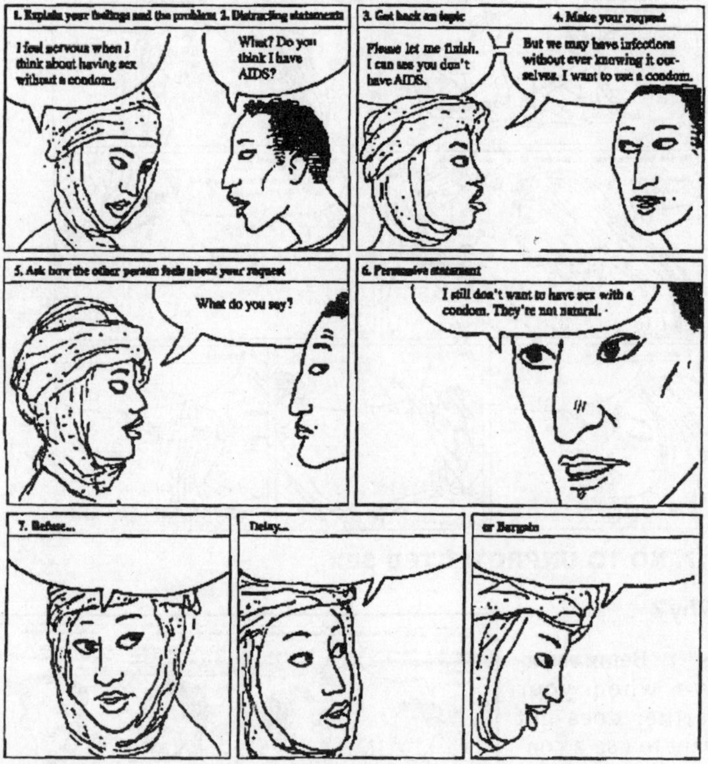
1. Explain your feelings and the problem
I feel nervous when I think about having sex without a condom.
2. Distracting statements
What? Do you think I have AIDS?
3. Get back on topic
Please let me finish. I can see you don't have AIDS.
4. Make your request
But we may have infections without ever knowing it ourselves. I want to use a condom.
5. Ask how the other person feels about your request
What do you say?
6. Persuasive statement
I still don't want to have sex with a condom. They're not natural.
7. Refuse...
Delay...
or Bargain

3.6. NO TO UNPROTECTED SEX

Why?

Being assertive when your partner does not want to use a condom is very important. The bottom line is "no sex without a condom".

How?

This situation will show you how to deal with a person who does not want to use a condom. This is done using the assertive skills you learned earlier.

"I'd be embarrassed to use a condom."

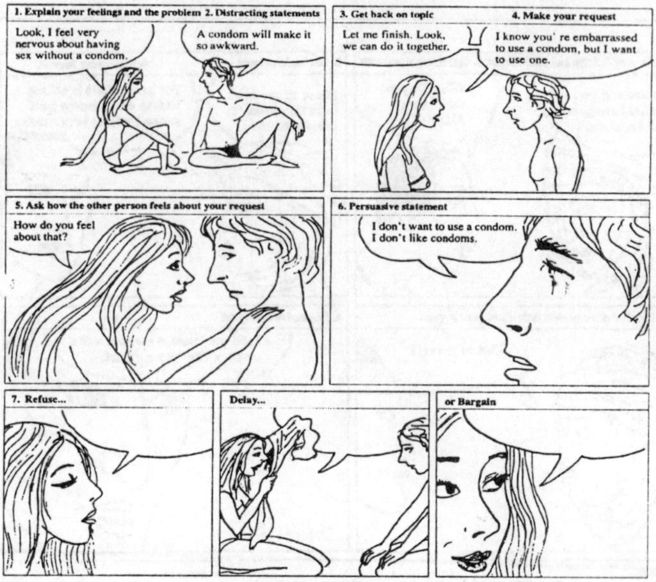
1. Explain your feelings and the problem
Look, I feel very nervous about having sex without a condom.
2. Distracting statements
A condom will make it so awkward.
3. Get back on topic
Let me finish. Look, we can do it together.
4. Make your request
I know you' re embarrassed to use a condom, but I want to use one.
5. Ask how the other person feels about your request
How do you feel about that?
6. Persuasive statement
I don't want to use a condom. I don't like condoms.
7. Refuse...
Delay...
or Bargain

3.7. NO TO UNPROTECTED SEX

Why?

Being assertive when your partner does not want to use a condom is very important. The bottom line is "no sex without a condom".

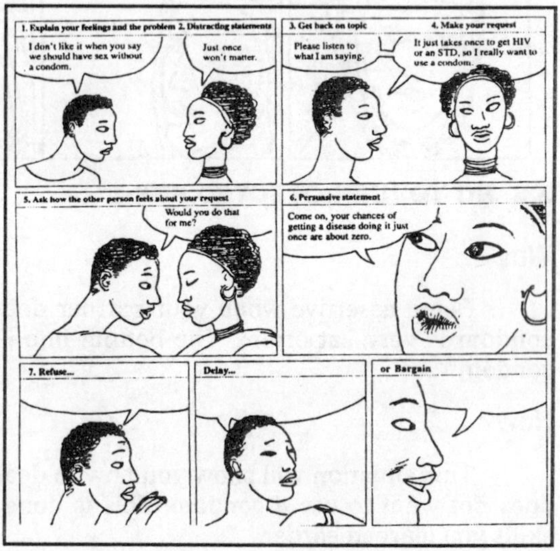
1. Explain your feelings and the problem
I don't like it when you say we should have sex without a condom.
2. Distracting statements
Just once won't matter.
3. Get back on topic
Please listen to what I am saying.
4. Make your request
It just takes once to get HIV or an STD, so I really want to use a condom.
5. Ask how the other person feels about your request
Would you do that for me?
6. Persuasive statement
Come on, your chances of getting a disease doing it just once are about zero.
7. Refuse...
Delay...
or Bargain

How?

This situation will show you how to deal with a person who does not want to use a condom. This is done using the assertive skills you learned earlier.

"I don't have a condom. Let's do it just this once."

Unit 4

Care and Support

4.1. WHO DISCRIMINATES?

Why?

When we don't give certain people the same rights and privileges as we do to others, we discriminate against them. How do we discriminate against people with HIV/AIDS? That is what this activity is about.

How?

1. Read the definition and examples of discrimination.
2. Read each discriminatory action against people with HIV/AIDS.
3. Complete the unfinished statement.
4. Answer the questions from "Teacher asks".

Discrimination

When we treat someone unjustly or unfavourably because of his/her race or religion, or because we believe he/she is ill, we discriminate against him/her.

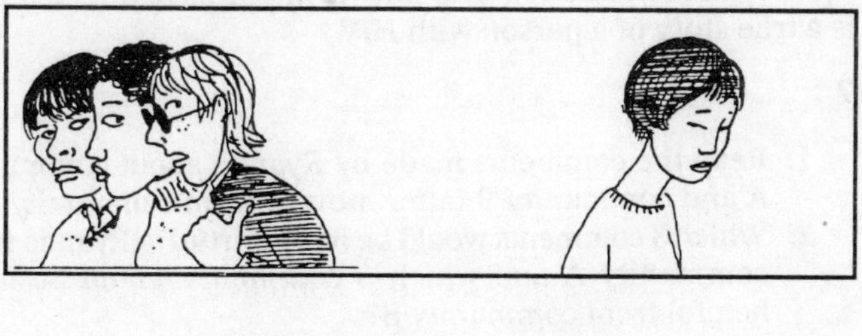

- *School discrimination*
  A person who has HIV is not allowed to attend school. ______________________
  This is wrong because: ______________________

- *The village banning*
  The Council will not allow people with AIDS to live in the village. ______________________
  This is wrong because: ______________________

- *Work in the fruit stand*
  Mancini, the owner of the fruit stand, won't allow Harsi, who has HIV, to work for him. This is wrong because: ______________________

- *A government decision*
  The government has decided not to allow people with HIV to enter the country. This will not stop AIDS because: ______________________

Teacher asks

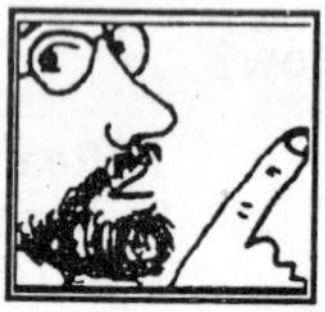

1. Why do people discriminate?
2. Why is it important not to discriminate?
3. What could you do if you heard discriminating remarks about a person with HIV or AIDS from someone in your community?

4.2. THE STORY OF TWO COMMUNITIES

Why?

If you have never been discriminated against, it is hard to understand what it feels like. In these two communities you are asked to imagine what Ryando felt and how it might have affected him. This is a true story of a person with HIV.

How?

1. Read the comments made by Ryando about community A and community B (after moving from community A).
2. Which 3 comments would be most hurtful to Ryando from community A and which 3 comments would be most helpful from community B?

Community A

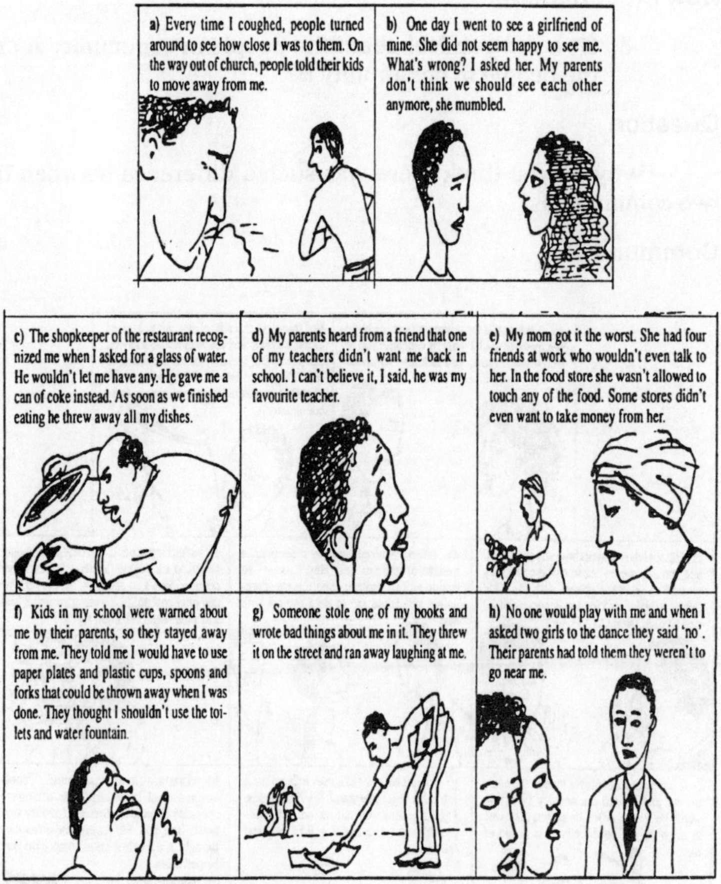
a) Every time I coughed, people turned around to see how close I was to them. On the way out of church, people told their kids to move away from me.
b) One day I went to see a girlfriend of mine. She did not seem happy to see me. What's wrong? I asked her. My parents don't think we should see each other anymore, she mumbled.
c) The shopkeeper of the restaurant recognized me when I asked for a glass of water. He wouldn't let me have any. He gave me a can of coke instead. As soon as we finished eating he threw away all my dishes.
d) My parents heard from a friend that one of my teachers didn't want me back in school. I can't believe it, I said, he was my favourite teacher.
e) My mom got it the worst. She had four friends at work who wouldn't even talk to her. In the food store she wasn't allowed to touch any of the food. Some stores didn't even want to take money from her.
f) Kids in my school were warned about me by their parents, so they stayed away from me. They told me I would have to use paper plates and plastic cups, spoons and forks that could be thrown away when I was done. They thought I shouldn't use the toilets and water fountain.
g) Someone stole one of my books and wrote bad things about me in it. They threw it on the street and ran away laughing at me.
h) No one would play with me and when I asked two girls to the dance they said 'no'. Their parents had told them they weren't to go near me.

Feelings about community A

Most hurtful	Reason why

THE STORY OF TWO COMMUNITIES

How? (continued)

3. How did you feel about the people in community A and the people in community B?

Question

Why do you think there was such a difference between the two communities?

Community B

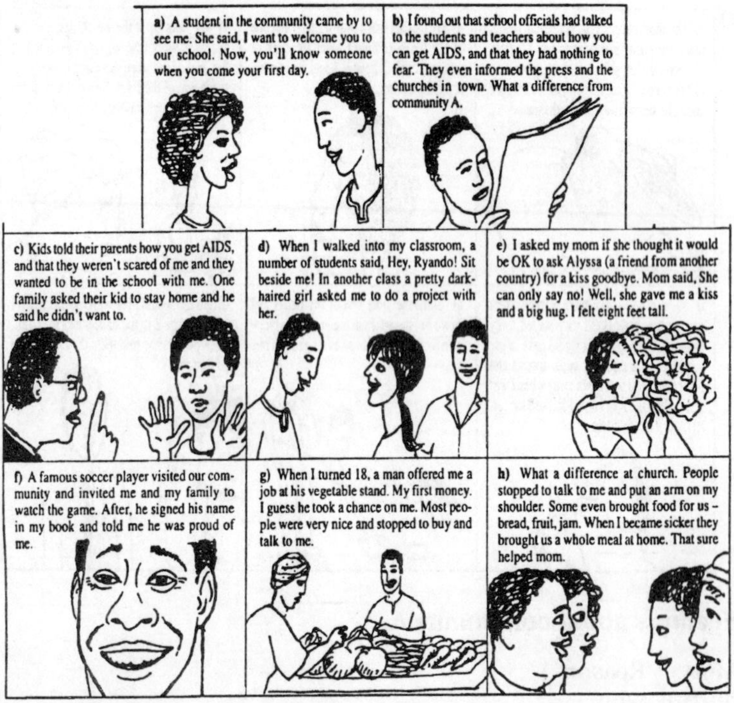

Feelings about community B

Most hurtful	Reason why
☐	______________________
☐	______________________
☐	______________________

4.3. WHY COMPASSION?

Why?

People who have compassion for others are very much needed. Compassion is understanding the pain of another person and wanting to do something to help.

How?

1. Read the "Reasons to show compassion to people living with AIDS".
2. Brainstorm five other reasons for being compassionate.
3. Decide on two reasons that are important for you and put a (√) beside them in the column "My two".
4. Answer the question in "Teacher asks".

Reasons to show compassion to people living with AIDS

My two	Reasons
	1. Everyone should be treated with understanding
	2. They are infected with a disease that has no cure
	3. It is good to think of someone other than yourself
	4. Other:
	5. Other:
	6. Other:
	7. Other:
	8. Other:
	9. Other:
	10. Other:

Teacher asks

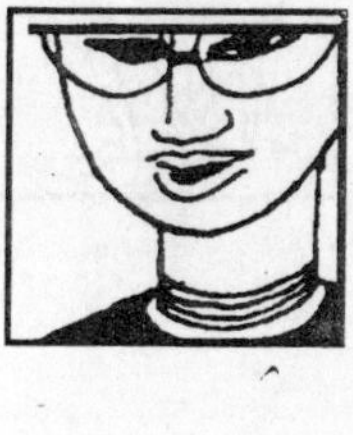

Why is it easy for some people to show compassion and more difficult for others?

4.4. WHAT COULD YOU DO?

Why?

Sometimes it is difficult to be compassionate because you don't know what you can do to help. In this activity you will learn ways to help two people whose stories are told below.

How?

1. Read the two stories below, keeping in mind how you might be able to help each person.
2. Then read the "Instructions" on the next page.

A mother with AIDS

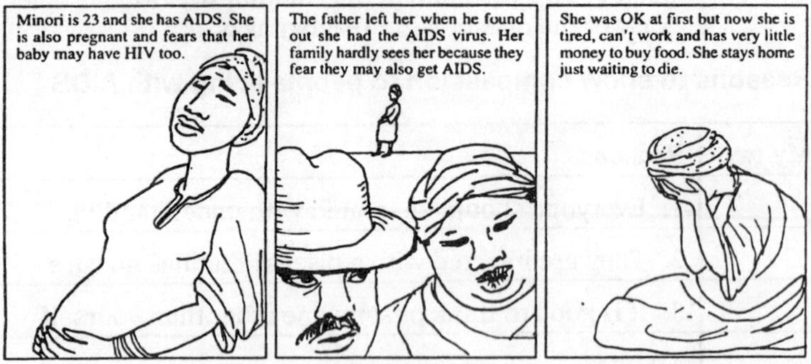
Minori is 23 and she has AIDS. She is also pregnant and fears that her baby may have HIV too.
The father left her when he found out she had the AIDS virus. Her family hardly sees her because they fear they may also get AIDS.
She was OK at first but now she is tired, can't work and has very little money to buy food. She stays home just waiting to die.

Dwari, a schoolmate

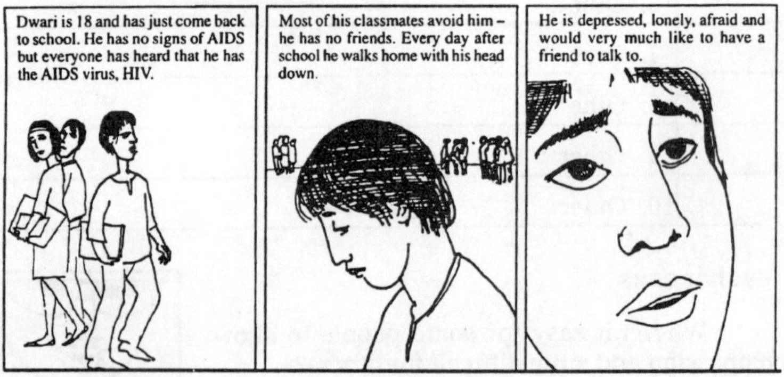

COULD YOU DO?

Instructions

1. Read all the ways you can help from the "The helping heart". Add any others that you can think of.
2. Select four things that you think you could do to help Minori and four for Dwari and put them in their hearts below.
3. Answer the question in "Teacher asks".

The helping heart

		Others:
• Say hello	• Ask them how you could help	
• Invite them for dinner	• Find others to give support	• ____________
• Just listen	• Get medicines	• ____________
• Leave them a letter	• Give a hug	• ____________
• Make or buy a meal	• Clean the house	• ____________
• Hold their hand	• Help other family members	• ____________
• Talk about the future	• Share emotions, laugh, cry	• ____________
• Celebrate special days	• Play games	• ____________

Minori's heart	Dwari's heart
• ____________	• ____________
• ____________	• ____________
• ____________	• ____________
• ____________	• ____________
• ____________	• ____________

Teacher asks

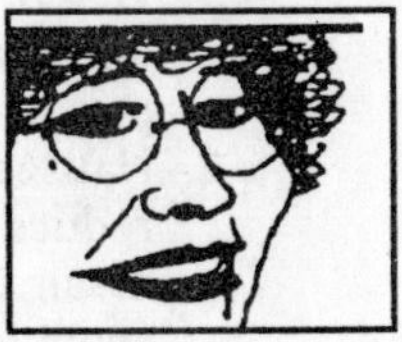

What would be most difficult for you if a friend or relative of yours had AIDS What would be most difficult for the person with AIDS?

4.5. HOW TO'S OF CAREGIVING

Why?

To be a caregiver for someone who has AIDS, means giving extra amounts of warmth and gentleness. Most people with AIDS are young adults who were alert, full of energy, and excited about life. For many, life has become full of fear, anger and fatigue. Many have lost friends, family, support from their community and hope, and they need others to care for them. A caregiver may need to be:

nurse, cook, food shopper, messenger, book reader, cleaner or listener. Overall, caregiving is being a friend and companion.

How?

Your teacher will give you instructions on how to do this activity.

A How to give emotional support

1. Share feelings - be honest and open.
2. Ask the person who is ill to talk about how he or she feels. Ask what they would like to do for themselves.
3. Say what you expect of the person who is ill and allow them to do the same.
4. Encourage him or her to do as much as possible for themselves. Do not do for the ill person what they can do for themselves.
5. Give support and praise when deserved.
6. Ask the person how they prefer to have things done, e.g. food preparation, cleaning.
7. When feelings of anger and crying occur, encourage them.
8. When care-giving, you need to look after yourself. You should take breaks and ask for help when needed.
9. The most common feelings are fear, anger, hopelessness, sadness, loneliness. Sit with the person. Let them know you are there to listen and talk to them.

B How to give physical support and care

1. Loss of appetite: Ask what they would like to eat and drink, when and how much. Eat with the ill person when possible.
2. Nausea and vomiting: Smaller meals with little fat may reduce vomiting. Encourage drinking liquids between meals if they can't eat. Notice when nausea occurs and avoid foods at this time. Use gloves to clean up vomit.
3. Lack of fluids: If a person has diarrhoea, vomiting and "sweats", they lose a lot of water. This could be very serious. If this happens, extra fluids (water, tea) should be given.
4. Weakness: Encourage activity (not strenuous). Have rest periods. Use a chair in the bath.
5. Skin problems: Change sleeping positions to avoid sores. Encourage short walks or sitting in a chair. Wash sores but use gloves if sores are open. Apply soothing lotions to dry skin.

6. Confusion and forgetting: AIDS and depression may affect the brain, causing confusion. Keep clocks and calendars and remind the person of the day, time and where they are. Make sure all safety precautions are taken for example, with loose rugs, stairs, medicines, sharp instruments etc.

Note

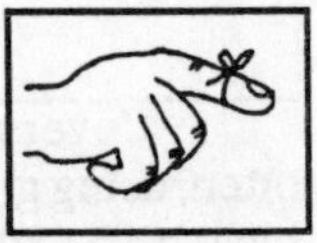

If you have difficulty or the condition looks serious, talk to a health worker or the health centre as soon as possible.

4.6. HOW TO KEEP YOURELF SAFE?

Garbage

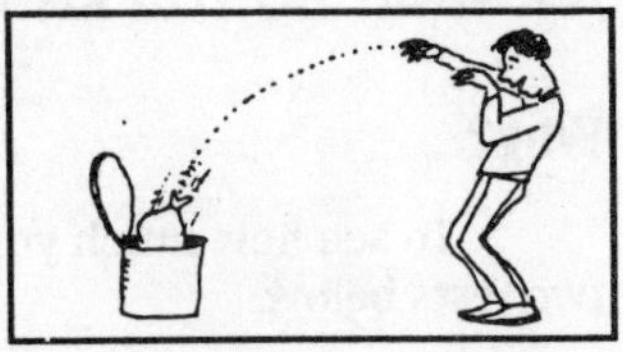

Things for cleaning (gloves and other soiled things) should be burned or placed in a double plastic bag. Tie the bag well before throwing out.

Laundry

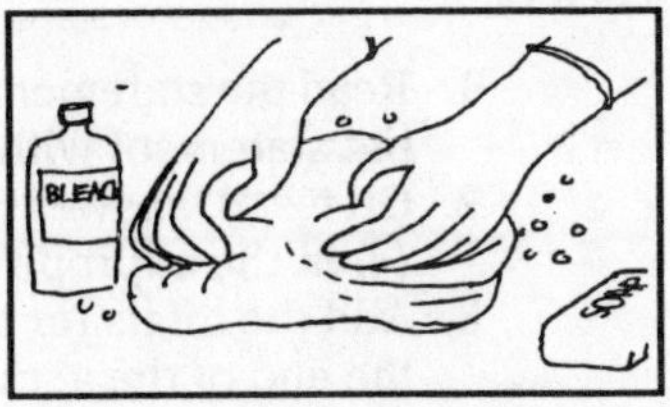

- If soiled with body fluids
  - wear gloves
  - use bleach and soap
  - keep separate from other laundry
- If not solied, wash as normal

Washing

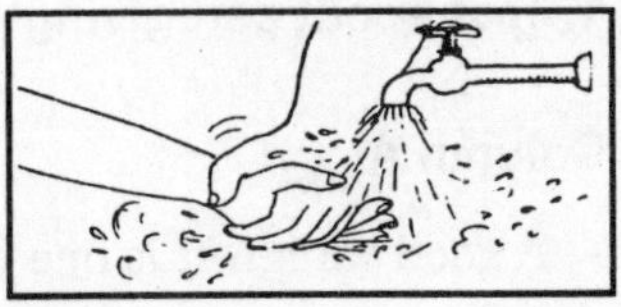

Wash your hands with warm, soapy water before and after contact with an ill person.

Instruments

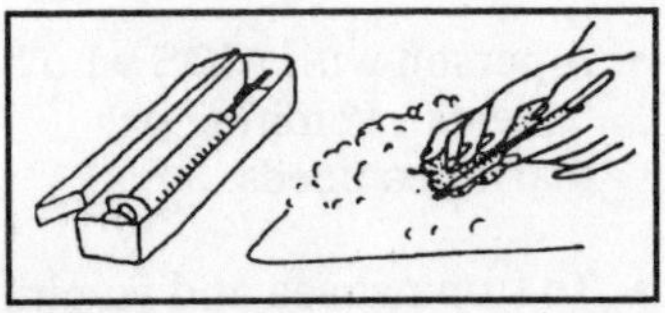

If injections are given, sterilize needles an syringes by boiling them; store them in plastic or metal box that won't puncture. Used disposable needles and syringes should be placed in thick cardboard, glass, plastic or metal containers and thrown away. Wash thermometers with soap and water.

Cleaning

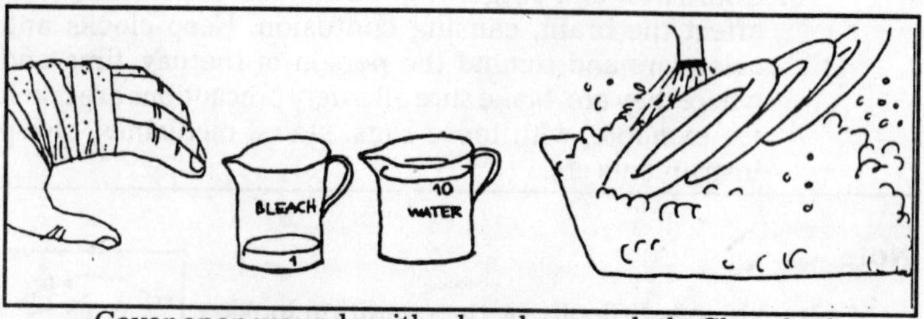

Cover open wounds with a bandage or cloth. Clean bathroom often, using gloves and bleach (1 part bleach to 10 parts water). Leave bleach 10 - 20 minutes before wiping up.

Also clean kitchen. Wash dishes with hot soapy water. Cloths used to clean the bathroom should not be used to clean the kitchen.

4.7. WHAT DO YOU KNOW?

Why?

To see how much you know about caregiving you can try the two tests below.

How?

1. Read the statements in test 1, column A, and try to match the statement with the correct answer in column B.
2. On test 2, answer true or false to each statement. Place a (√) in the appropriate box.
3. Add the totals for tests 1 and 2 and find your "Rating" at the end of the activity.

1. Test about caregiving - matching

Column A		Column B
• A good caregiver is one who is a...	☐	a) Angry or cry
• A person with AIDS who has "sweats", vomiting or diarrhoea needs...	☐	b) Look after yourself
• To stop nausea and vomiting it is best to give....	☐	c) Extra fluids
• For a person who is in bed a lot you should...	☐	d) Friend and companion

• As a good caregiver you should also...	☐	e) Really listen
• You should encourage people who are sad and depressed to express their feelings if they become...	☐	f) Small meals with little fat
• People who are ill need to do...	☐	g) What they can for themselves
• The most important skill in being a good caregiver is to...	☐	h) Change their sleeping position

2. True - False statements

T	F	
☐	☐	1. Latex or rubber gloves should be used when touching body fluids.
☐	☐	2. Injecting needles should be put in a plastic bag.
☐	☐	3. Thermometers can be used more than once without washing.
☐	☐	4. The most important thing in looking after yourself is to wash your hands with soap and warm water.
☐	☐	5. There have been no HIV infections from living in the same house as a person who has HIV or AIDS.
☐	☐	6. Soiled things should be put in a paper bag and then put in the garbage.
☐	☐	7. It is very important to cover sores, cuts and rashes.
☐	☐	8. You should wash the bathroom with bleach solution that is 1 part bleach to 20 parts water.

Test I score + Test 2 score = Total score

☐ ☐ ☐

Rating	
13-16 points	Super memory
9 - 12 points	A good caregiver
5 - 8 points	Try to do better next time!
1 - 4 points	You still have a lot to learn !

4.8. SUPPORT FOR RESPONSIBLE BEHAVIOUR

Why?

Young people sometimes take risks with their health and safety. With AIDS around this can be dangerous. Young people who make the right decisions to delay sex, to use a condom or to be tolerant and compassionate to people with AIDS, need the support of their friends.

How?

1. Read one of the stories below.
2. Decide what you could do to give the main person in your story support for a healthy decision.
3. Write two or three statements of support for each story. You may be asked to role-play your responses.
4. Answer the questions for each story in "Teacher asks".

Story A- A decision not to have sex

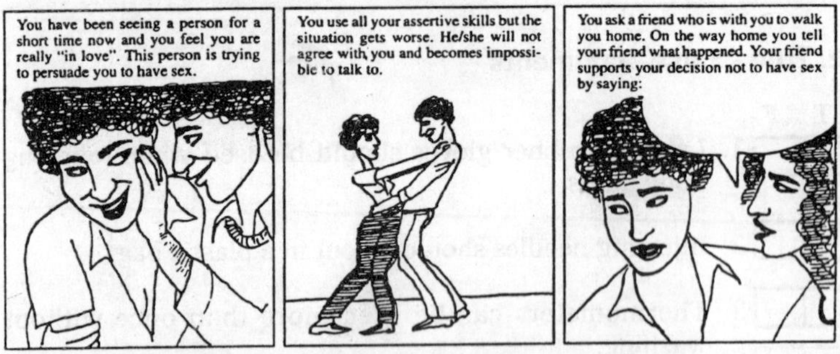
You have been seeing a person for a short time now and you feel you are really "in love". This person is trying to persuade you to have sex.
You use all your assertive skills but the situation gets worse. He/she will not agree with you and becomes impossible to talk to.
You ask a friend who is with you to walk you home. On the way home you tell your friend what happened. Your friend supports your decision not to have sex by saying:

Story B-No sex without a condom

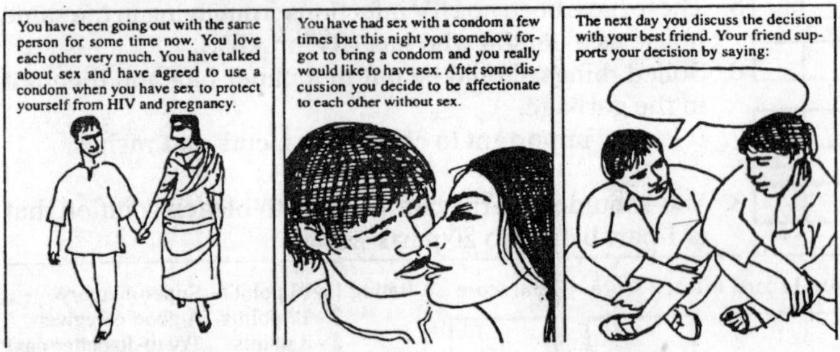
You have been going out with the same person for some time now. You love each other very much. You have talked about sex and have agreed to use a condom when you have sex to protect yourself from HIV and pregnancy.
You have had sex with a condom a few times but this night you somehow forgot to bring a condom and you really would like to have sex. After some discussion you decide to be affectionate to each other without sex.
The next day you discuss the decision with your best friend. Your friend supports your decision by saying:

SUPPORT FOR RESPONSIBLE BEHAVIOUR

Story C - To go to the candy store or not

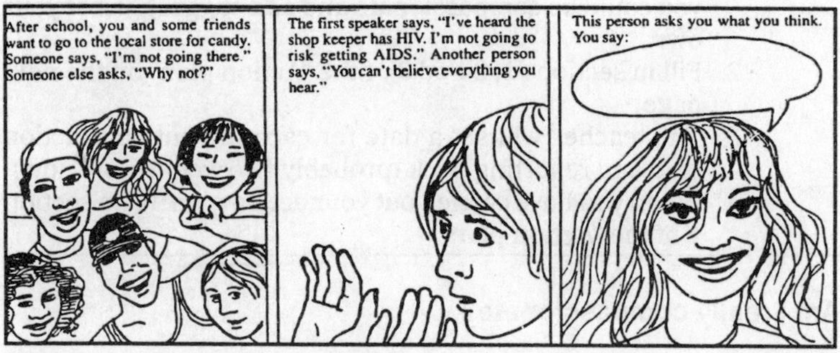
After school, you and some friends want to go to the local store for candy. Someone says, "I'm not going there." Someone else asks, "Why not?"
The first speaker says, "I've heard the shop keeper has HIV. I'm not going to risk getting AIDS." Another person says, "You can't believe everything you hear."
This person asks you what you think. You say:

Story D-Who do you support

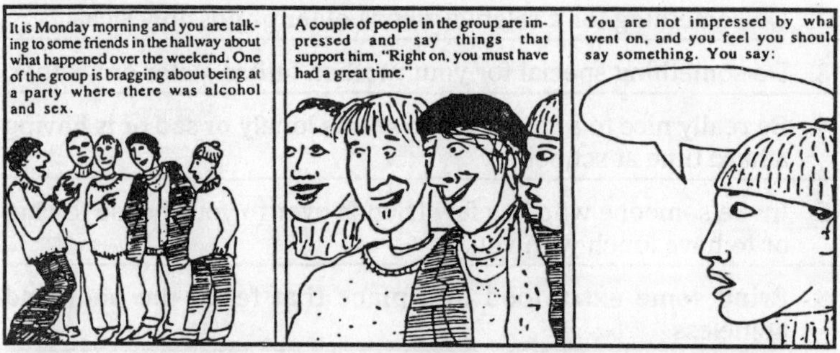
It is Monday morning and you are talking to some friends in the hallway about what happened over the weekend. One of the group is bragging about being at a party where there was alcohol and sex.
A couple of people in the group are impressed and say things that support him, "Right on, you must have had a great time."
You are not impressed by wha went on, and you feel you shoul say something. You say:

Teacher asks

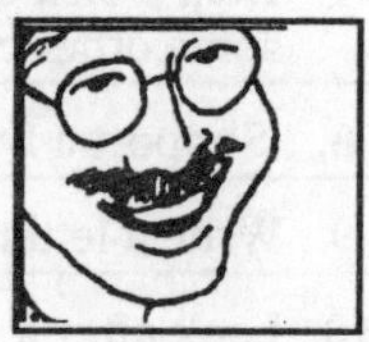

1. Why do many young people feel it is not "cool" to support healthy decisions?
2. What difficulties might you have if you support healthy behaviours?
3. How might you overcome these problems?

4.9. COMPASSION, TOLERANCE AND SUPPORT

Why?

Knowing how to be compassionate, tolerant and supportive will mean little to you unless you actually practise these behaviours in everyday situations.

How?

1. Select someone, or a group of people that you think needs support or compassion. Look at the list below, of ways you could be compassionate and add suggestions of your own.
2. Fill in sections 1, 2 and 3 of the "Action plan" on the next page.
3. The teacher will set a date for carrying out your action plan and reporting back (probably two weeks from now).
4. When you have carried out your action plan, fill in section 4 of the "Action plan"

Am I really compassionate?

1. Visit a hospital to talk to someone or to bring them flowers, etc.
2. Do something for a relative who is older or possibly sick.
3. Do something special for your mother, father, sister or brother.
4. Be really nice to a student who seems lonely or sad or is having a hard time at school.
5. Invite someone who has few friends over to your house to chat or to have lunch with you.
6. Bring some extra food to a place that feeds the poor and homeless.
7. Help a sick or elderly neighbour fetch water or firewood or do some other chore.
8. Support a friend who is having difficulties in their life.
9. Write a letter to someone who is sick or lonely.
10. Look after a baby, free of charge, for someone who is having a hard time.

COMPASSION, TOLERANCE AND SUPPORT

Action plan

1. My selection ________________________________

____

____

____

____

____

2. Reasons for my selection ______________________

____

____

____

____

3. What I could do: ______________________

a) ______________________________________

b) ______________________________________

c) ______________________________________

____

4. Summary of what happened and my feelings

____

____

____

____

PART-III

Teachers' Guide

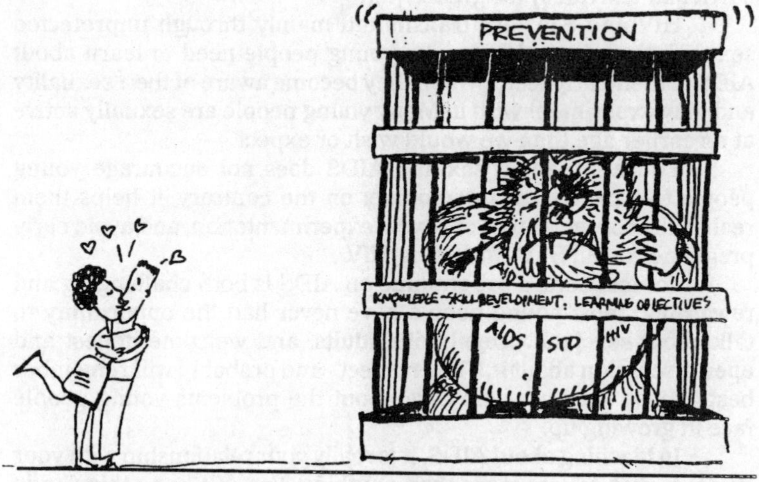

INTRODUCTION

Dear teacher....

This guide has been developed to help you prepare and teach a programme on AIDS.

AIDS (Acquired Immune Deficiency Syndrome) has become a problem in our country: to date, some [give here latest figures] women and men have died from AIDS, another [...] are sick, and an estimated [...] are infected with HIV (Human Immunodeficiency Virus), the virus that causes AIDS. Sexually transmitted diseases (STD) are very common: [give figures that show that STD are a serious problem, particularly for youth].

As educators and parents, we can do much to save our students and families from AIDS: we can explain to them how to protect themselves from infection with HIV and other STD. There is no cure yet for AIDS, but we can easily avoid infection with HIV and STD.

Much is done in our country to provide information on AIDS and STD [mention posters, TVradio programmes, reports in the press, etc.]. Health personnel are trained to care for people with AIDS in health centres and hospitals, and blood for transfusions is being tested [add information to allay fears of casual transmission].

Young people need to know how to protect themselves from HIV and STD. To reach all the young people in school, AIDS education has been integrated into [give here the subject(s) or extra-curricular activities] for grades [...].

HIV and STD are transmitted mainly through unprotected sexual intercourse: that is why young people need to learn about AIDS in their early teens, when they become aware of their sexuality and may experiment with it. Many young people are sexually active at an earlier age than we would wish or expect.

Education about sex and AIDS does not encourage young people to have sexual intercourse: on the contrary, it helps them realize the consequences of sexual experimentation, and avoid early pregnancies and STD, including HIV.

For teachers, a programme on AIDS is both challenging and rewarding: most young people have never had the opportunity to talk about sex [and drugs] with adults, and welcome honest and open discussion about it. They respect - and probably will remember best - those teachers who care about the problems young people face in growing up.

In teaching about AIDS, it is really your relationship with your students that counts more than anything else. We hope this Guide will be useful in providing factual information and the required teaching methods.

Information is provided for you on the following topics:

1. The programme

This section presents the rationale for the programme; the four units of the programme and the objectives of each unit; and a description of the student activities that are available for each unit.

2. Teaching methods

Since this programme is based mainly on participatory methods, it is important to know the basic ways of getting students involved. Seven different methods are discussed in this section.

3. The classroom atmosphere

Sexuality education should be conducted in an atmosphere that promotes openness and acceptance. This section provides information on: the reactions of students to discussions about sexuality; rules to develop classroom atmosphere; how to deal with special problems; and how to help the student who might be anxious about HIV/AIDS/STD.

4. Peer leaders [if applicable]

Teachers are encouraged to use peer leaders as part of this programme. This section discusses: the functions of peer leaders; why it is important to use peer leaders; how to select peer leaders; and what peer leaders need to know.

5. Participation of parents and family members

The support of parents for HIV/AIDS/STD education is very important to the success of a programme. This section discusses: parent letters; parent meetings; parent/student activities; and advantages of parent involvement.

6. Test items for student evaluation

This section presents test items for students, that match the curriculum.

7. Questions on HIV/AIDS/STD

This section is very important. Teachers need to be very familiar with the facts about HIV/ AIDS/STD so that they can provide accurate information in response to questions that concerned young people may ask. A thorough review of the questions and answers in this section should be completed before starting the programme.

Teachers' guide to the student activities

For each student activity suggested for use in your classroom, there is guidance on:

- How to do that activity; answers to the questions or activities;
- Special concerns about the activity (if applicable);
- Use of peer leaders; parent involvement (if used);
- Additional information or preparation teachers might need.

THE PROGRAMME

The goal of AIDS education is to promote behaviour that prevents the transmission of HIV/STD. Learning the behavioural skills that are needed for prevention forms the major content of this curriculum.

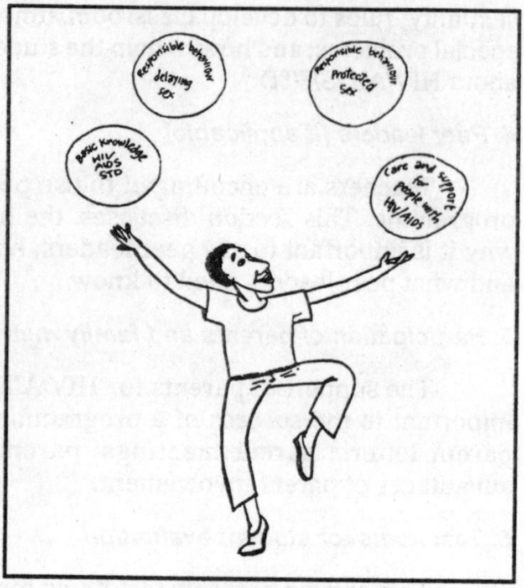

As you can see, the curriculum is concerned more with the development of skills for responsible behaviour than with knowledge about AIDS.

The programme is based on the observation that biomedical information on the disease is not enough to convince people, including young people, to adopt healthy behaviour that prevents HIV/STD. What is needed is the motivation to act and skills to translate knowledge into practice.

Infection with HIV/STD occurs in specific risk situations or scenarios: a girl is pressured by her boyfriend into having sex, [...give examples from the situation assessment study]. Young people in these situations need to have the knowledge and skills to respond adequately, for example, how to say "no" or how to propose alternatives.

Through the achievement of a set of learning objectives, the curriculum aims to increase knowledge and to develop skills, positive attitudes and motivation.

Knowledge

Information that will help students decide what behaviours are healthy and responsible includes: ways HIV/STD are transmitted and not transmitted; the stages of the disease especially the long asymptomatic period of HIV; personal vulnerability to HIV/STD; means of protection from HIV/STD; sources of help, if needed; and how to care for people in the family who have AIDS.

Skill development

The skills relevant to HIV/AIDS preventive behaviours are: self-awareness; decision making; to have sex; negotiation skills to ensure protected sex; and practical skills for effective condom use. These skills are best taught through rehearsal or role-play of real-life situations that might put young people at risk for HIV/STD.

Attitudes

Attitudes to HIV/AIDS/STD include: positive attitudes towards delaying sex, personal responsibility, condoms as a means of protection; social attitudes such as confronting prejudice, being supportive, tolerant and compassionate towards people with HIV and AIDS; and sensible attitudes about drug use, multiple partners and voilent abusive relationships.

Motivational supports

Even a well-informed and skilled person needs to be motivated to initiate and maintain safe practices. A realistic perception of the student's own risk and of the benefits of adopting preventive behaviour is closely related to motivation. Peer reinforcement and support for healthy actions is crucial, as peer norms are powerful motivators of young people's behaviour. Programmes that use peer leaders are effective because peers are likely to be more familiar with youth language and culture. Parents can also motivate and reinforce the objectives of the programme and should be encouraged to play a part in their child's sexuality education.

Learning objectives

The programme has been designed so that at the end of it, students will be able to: [present here the list of all the learning objectives].

The programme consists of four units:

Unit 1

Basic knowledge of HIV/AIDS/STD

This unit presents the basic information on HIV, AIDS, STD; how HIV/STD are transmitted; how they are not transmitted; methods of protection from HIV/STD; difference between HIV and AIDS; sources of help. Note that this unit takes about 25% of the curriculum. Objectives [...] are covered in this unit.

Unit 2

Responsible behaviour: delaying sex

Students, particularly at early ages, should be encouraged not to have sexual intercourse. Delaying sex to an older age usually results in more mature decisions about contraception and protected sex. Students need to discuss the reasons and supports for delaying sexual intercourse, and learn how to resist pressures for unwanted sex. Assertive communication skills should be learned through role-play of real-life situations that young people may encounter. They may also learn that affection can be shown in ways other than sexual intercourse. Objectives [...] are covered in this unit.

Unit 3

Responsible behaviour: protected sex

Some, perhaps many students may already be sexually active at the time they learn about AIDS in this programme. Others will need to know how to protect themselves in the future when they will be sexually active. Using condom every time one has sexual intercours is a very effective way to avoid infection with HIV/STD. Teaching students about condom. does not mean encouraging them to have sex young people are exposed to information about condoms through a variety of sources (friends, media, condoms displayed in shops etc.), and need to have information and skills on how to use condoms correctly. Objective [...] are covered in this unit.

Units 2 and 3 on responsible behaviour should take approximately 50% of the total classroom] time given to the AIDS/STD programme. This is because prevention through responsible behaviour is the most important part of the programme, and the learning of skills tend to be time-consuming.

Unit 4

Care and support for people with HIV/AIDS

Many young people will come in contact with people with HIV and AIDS, perhaps in their own family and community. They need to learn tolerance, compassion, and ways to care for and support these people. Unit 4 covers objectives [...] and will take approximate 125% of the programme.

The programme activities

For each unit, a number of student activities have been developed (see the set of students' activities). For each student activity, this book gives you detailed guidance for its use in the classroom.

Active learning by students is a major objective of the programme: many classroom activities involve participation by students, while some are mostly informational. [list here the activities of each unit with a rationale and a short description].

You may find some of the activities controversial, or the language too explicit for young people.

[Identify those activities that teachers may have difficulty in accepting, and give the rationale:].

Activity 6 - unit 2, for example, presents nonpenetrative sex as a safer alternative to sexual intercourse. It is important that young people are aware that penetrative sexual intercourse is not the only way to obtain sexual pleasure...

Unit 3 is about protected sex and condoms. Although the curriculum stresses that delaying sexual intercourse is a very safe way of avoiding HIV and STD while young, we know that virtually all will become sexually active at some point in their lives. We have to equip our young people to protect themselves from infection when they become sexually active. Evaluation of sex education programmes has shown that knowledge of and access to contraceptives (like the condom) does not lead to increased sexual activity in young people. We should not forget that many of our students are already sexually active, and the message of "delaying sex" is of little relevance to them. Condoms also protect girls from unwanted pregnancies, which are a major problem in our country.

Using condoms for extra-marital relationships is also a form of responsible behaviour, because it protects the wife and the children from becoming infected: too many women, who themselves are faithful, are infected by their husbands who have other relationships, and often find out they are infected with HIV when their children get sick and die of AIDS.

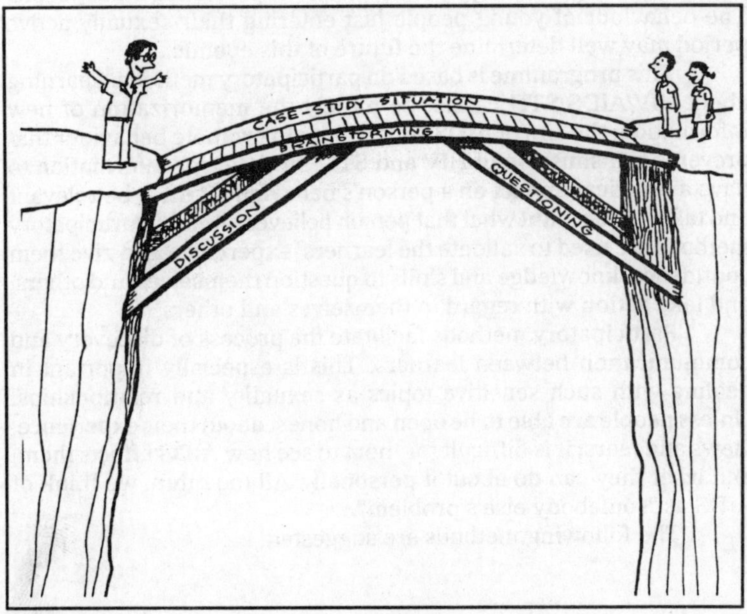

TEACHING METHODS

Teaching teenagers about HIV/AIDS/STD requires a frank and explicit discussion of sexuality, modes of transmission and methods of protection. Many may be embarrassed about discussing sexuality and related issues. Fortunately, no one has died of embarrassment and we really have no choice, if we want to protect our children from a deadly disease.

Don't pretend you are not embarrassed when in fact you are. Admit that it is difficult for you, but that it is too important not to talk about it. Start by saying it often is an embarrassing topic and when people are uncomfortable they laugh, make jokes or do other things to cover up their nervousness. This is very effective for the purposes of class control.

Remember that the students in the classroom have different experiences in relation to sex: some are sexually active, others are not; some may be victims of sexual abuse; some had the opportunity to learn about sexuality with a caring adult or older sibling, others have only "street" knowledge; some may have sex to pay for school fees and uniforms. Your language should not be judgemental: this would make some students feel excluded, and therefore, not interested in prevention.

Present sexuality in positive terms. Then HIV/AIDS/ STD can be put in the proper context. Explain that prevention of HIV is not just a matter of protecting yourself but also of protecting other people. The behaviour of young people just entering their sexually active period may well determine the future of this epemlc.

This programme is based on participatory methods. Learning about HIV/AIDS/STD cannot be merely the memorization of new information: the aim of AIDS education is to promote behaviour that prevents transmission of HIV and STD. In order for information to have a practical impact on a person's behaviour, it must be relevant and take into account what that person believes already. Participatory methods are used to validate the learners' experience and give them confidence, knowledge and skills to question themselves and others, and take action with regard to themselves and others.

Participatory methods facilitate the process of discovery and communication between learners. This is especially important in dealing with such sensitive topics as sexuality and relationships. Unless people are able to be open and honest about their experience, views and fears, it is difficult for them to see how AIDS affects them, and what they can do about it personally. All too often, we think of AIDS as "somebody else's problem".

The following methods are suggested:

Discussion

Discussions can be held with the whole class but they work best when held in small groups. Group discussion stimulates free exchange of ideas, and helps individuals to clarify ideas, feelings, and attitudes. Discussion works very well if it follows some kind of "trigger", e.g. a case study, a story.

Questioning

When conducting a group discussion, teachers should be aware of the impact of "putting down" a student's response. By not accepting responses in a positive way, the teacher may discourage students from answering further questions. The pacing of questions is also important. Students should be given time to think about a response but questions should be rapid enough to keep the pace of the class lively. Try not to ask questions that result in a one word response, e.g. "yes" or "no". Open, clarifying questions should be asked so as to encourage students to talk.

Brainstorming

Brainstorming is a technique in which every student's response that applies to the topic is acceptable. It is important to not evaluate ideas but to accept everything and to record each idea on the blackboard or a piece of paper. Students need to know that they will not be required to justify or explain any answer. After the period of time for brainstorming, (which should not be too long), time for reflection or prioritizing of the list should be allowed. Brainstorming is effective for:

- Sensitive and controversial issues that need to be explored.
- Encouraging students who are hesitant to enter a discussion.
- Gathering a lot of ideas quickly.

Role-play

Role-play involves presenting a short spontaneous play which describes possible real-life situations. In role-play, we imitate someone else's character. This is often easier than having to express our own ideas and feelings.

Role-play is a very effective technique but also a difficult one to master. The following points may help you to make this method more effective:

- Select volunteers, or students who are outgoing and energetic.
- Involve yourself in one of the main roles.

- Give students some lines or a script to get them started.
- Use "props" - hats, cards with names on, wigs, etc.
- Use humour, if possible.
- Pair all students in the class and have each one play a role, e.g. a father and a son. This will eliminate embarrassment of being in front of the class.

Case study/situation

A case study is a fictional story that allows students to make decisions about how the person should act or respond and what the consequences of their actions might be. Case studies allow the students to discuss someone else's behaviour and, therefore, to avoid revealing personal experiences that might be embarrassing to them.

The case study can be open-ended, that is, the ending of the story may be missing. It is up to the students to decide on all possible conclusions and the consequences and to finally decide on what would be the best ending for the situation.

Group work

Many of the activities contained in the units suggest small group work. Here are some teaching points if you decide to try small group work.

- It is best to start with pairs or groups of three or four. This tends to be less threatening to students. As confidence builds, you can make the groups larger.
- Try to vary the methods used for forming groups as much as possible and make sure that students frequently work with different class members. You decide on the groups. It is best not to let students form their own groups. Those students who are left out (not selected) will feel inferior and not wanted.
- Try giving group responsibilities, e.g. recorder, encourager, keeping the group on their task, time keeper, presenter of group's work, etc.
- Emphasize a "sink or swim together" attitude. All members must contribute to the assigned task. The group's success depends on the individual contribution of each member.
- It may be important at times to use groups where the sexes are separated rather than mixed.

Other methods

Story telling is a traditional method of providing information and discussion topics. Situations in the student activities can be told in a story-telling format using the local culture as a base for the story.

Fables are stories that have been told to explain how people can put themselves in danger by acting a certain way. Fables often involve animals as the characters and, therefore, present a message without students feeling badly about their behaviour. The stories can be developed to contain health messages about AIDS and can be followed by a discussion on what was learned and how things could be changed to make it better.

Expressing health messages or feelings about AIDS through music, dance or poetry can be very effective. Use tunes that are known locally and have students put their own words to them. Use dances that everyone knows and put words to them. The whole group can participate in writing the words.

You can develop your role-plays (from the student activities) into full plays which you can then act for parents or students from other schools or other classrooms. At the end of the play, the messages can be discussed with the audience.

Puppets can do things that actors may find difficult to express because of cultural reasons. The audience can ask the puppets questions after the show. This is particularly effective with AIDS issues which can be either embarrassing or difficult to discuss openly.

Methods for large classes

Teachers coping with very large classes of students are unable to interact with students to the point where they are able to hold frank, open discussions. Where there are very large classes, the chalk board is the main teaching aid. In this situation, the teacher can successfully teach facts about AIDS using usual classroom techniques. However, information and activities which involve the students in examining behaviour and experiences have to be organized largely with the participation of the students. Students can be divided into groups, and helped by peer leaders (see section 4).

Following the factual lessons about AIDS, students may carry out group projects, and report back in various ways, e.g. making charts, illustrations, giving reports through talks, role play, drama, etc. Groups report their findings to each other and display their work. Possible topics and tasks:

- What we know about HIV/AIDS/STD.
- What our families know about HIV/AIDS/STD.
- What the community knows about HIV/AIDS/STD.
- What is done at the health centre about people with HIV/AIDS/STD: interview with nurses/doctors.
- Group identifies and collects existing materials, posters, radio/TV plays, to inform people about HIV/ AIDS/STD.
- Group finds out which individuals, groups or organizations exist in the community for giving

information. Each group holds a meeting with one of the identified persons/organizations.

- Group carries out opinion survey and displays results.
- Group identifies the main recreational activities of peers.
- Group identifies behaviours which could cause the spread of AIDS among different age groups.
- Groups hold meetings to explain AIDS.
- Groups arrange debates/competitions/social events.
- Groups write and act various plays to illustrate the danger of HIV/AIDS in the community.

At the conclusion of such projects, the teacher can arrange for a special guest to be present at the display of findings.

Often at the end of such projects, students can go on to develop other themes which further investigate their social circumstances and involve them in exposing drug and alcohol abuse etc. using the same approaches.

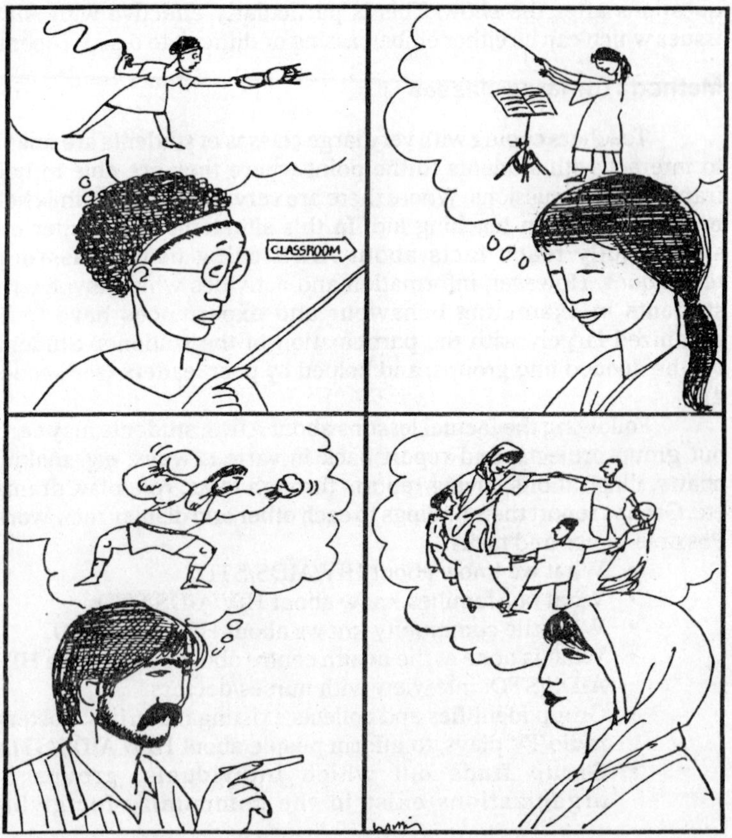

THE CLASSROOM ATMOSPHERE

Students may react to this programme in different ways. They may:

- Ask baiting questions (to try to embarrass you).
- Remain silent because of embarrassment.
- Shock or try to amuse by describing sexually explicit behaviours.
- Ask very personal questions about your private life.
- Make comments that open themselves to peer ridicule or criticism.

To deal with these situations it is important to set class rules. These must be very clear to the students before you start. You can have students develop their own rules or you can start with a list and discuss with the students if they are fair and why they are important. A suggested list might be:

- Students are expected to treat each other in a positive way and be considerate of each other's feelings.
- Students are not to discuss personal matters that were raised during the lesson with others outside of the classroom.
- Students should avoid interrupting each other.
- Students should listen to each other and respect each other's opinions.
- Both students and teachers have a "right-to-pass" if questions are too personal.
- No put-downs - no matter how much you disagree with the person you do not laugh, make a joke about them or use language that would make that person feel inferior.
- Students may be offered the possibility of putting their questions anonymously to the teacher.
- Many times students laugh and giggle about sex. This should be allowed in the beginning, as it lowers the barriers when discussing sexuality.

Strategies to deal with special problems

The following strategies might be used to deal with personal questions, explicit language and inappropriate behaviour.

- Respond to statements that put down or reinforce stereotypes (for example, statements that imply that some groups of people are responsible for the AIDS epidemic) by discussing the implications of such statements.

- Be assertive in dealing with difficult situations for example, "That topic is not appropriate for this class. If you would like to discuss it, I'd be happy to talk to you after class".
- Avoid being overly critical about answers - so that students will be encouraged to express their opinions openly and honestly.
- Present both sides of a controversial issue. Avoid making value judgements.
- It might be important to separate males and females in group activities that might be embarrassing to the students or where separated groups may function more efficiently.

Helping the anxious student

- It is helpful to think ahead of how you might respond to students in the class who believe they may have been exposed to HIV or have an STD. It is important that you behave in such a way that students who are worried will feel comfortable seeking your advice.
- Your responsibility in teaching an HIV/AIDS/STD programme includes learning in advance what help and services are available in your community.
- Listen to the student who approaches you, without imposing your values, moral judgements or opinions. Do not ask leading or suggestive questions about his or her behaviour.
- Convey your concern for the student's health and when appropriate, tell the student that you know of services that can help him/her. Offer to start the process by contacting the one the student chooses.
- Continue your support by confidentially asking the student from time to time if he or she needs more information, has taken any action, or is still concerned about anything related to your conversation.

PEER LEADERS

Why peer leaders

Young people listen more attentively and accept messages from respected peers more readily than from a teacher. This is especially true in areas of health, safety and sexuality. Some students are influential in that they set the group norms and function as models for the group. They can become peer leaders. Peer leaders provide assistance to the teacher which allows him/her to spend more time on preparation, individual attention nal rlS room mana,vement.

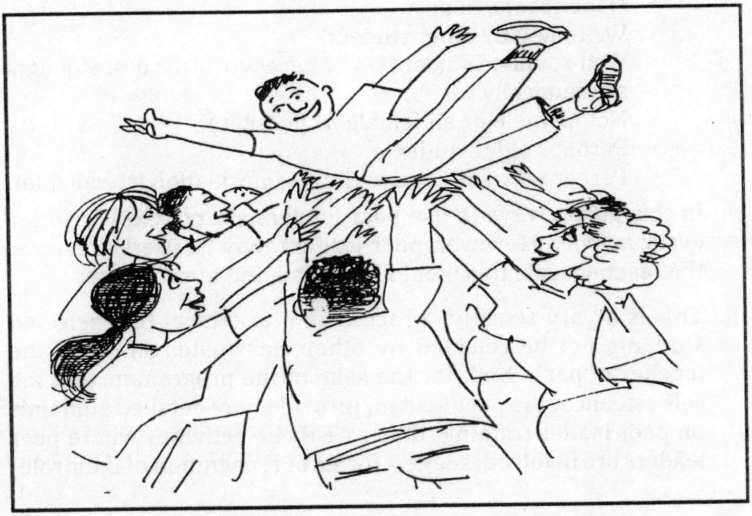

Who is a peer leader

A peer leader is a person who helps the teacher in many ways:

- Helps in classroom management, e.g. handing out activity sheets, etc.
- Helps in demonstrations, e.g. using a condom
- Helps in role-plays, e.g. being assertive
- Leads a class team, e.g. during a quiz
- Reads stories, questions, answers to activities
- Volunteers answers to activities
- Leads a small group
- Reports findings of small groups
- Models appropriate behaviour, e.g. is assertive
- Carries out certain activities and reports back, e.g. buying a condom
- Takes polls, e.g. when teacher wants to know how many answered"yes".
- Draws diagrams on the blackboard.

Selection of peer leader(s)

Peer leaders may be selected by their own peers. Otherwise, select from the class individuals who are:

- Considered as opinion-leaders by the other students.
- Concerned about the welfare of their peers.
- Able to listen to others.
- Self-confident.

- Dependable, honest.
- Well-liked by other students
- Well-rounded students - not necessarily the best students academically.
- Not all male or all female (if possible).
- Perhaps older students.
- Perhaps sexually active (if this information is available).

In this guide, ways to use peer leaders are not explained for every activity. However, peer leaders may be used whenever the teacher feels this would be useful and appropriate.

This is a very sensitive process as it is critical that selected students not be rejected by other classmates as being the teacher's "pet" - both for the sake of the programme and the self-esteem of the peer leaders [provide here detailed guidance on peer leader training, illustrate those activities where peer leaders are involved, suggest forms of recognition of their role]

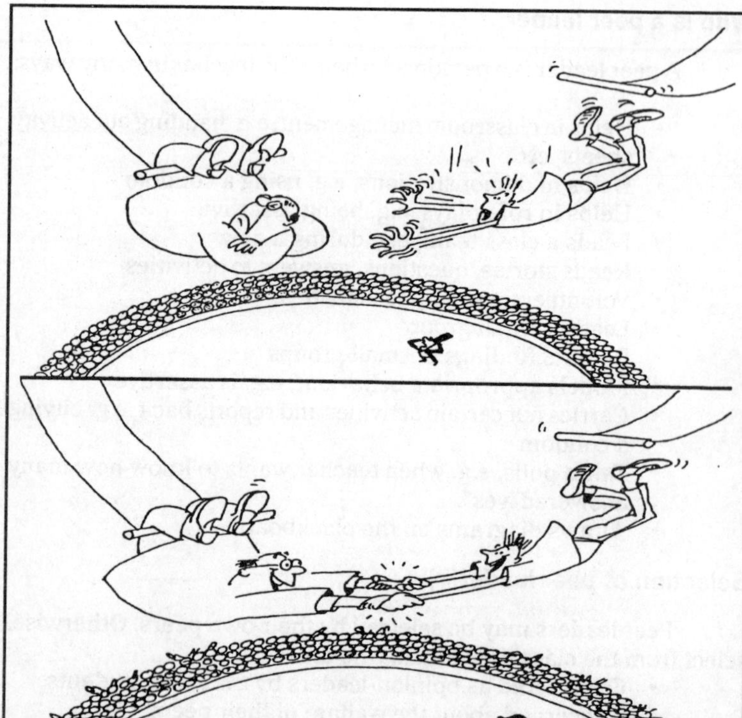

PARTICIPATION OF PARENTS AND FAMILY MEMBERS

It is important to involve parents in the programme: families have an important role in the development of personal and ethical values in our students. Most parents recognize the threat posed by AIDS, and are in favour of school education for prevention. Some of them find it difficult to discuss sexuality with their children, and are happy if the school takes on the responsibility. However, they may have reservations about some parts of the programme.

Parents often need to learn about AIDS themselves, and the school programme may provide the opportunity for parents, and other members of the family, to obtain accurate information, and to dispel myths or rumours about AIDS that circulate in the community.

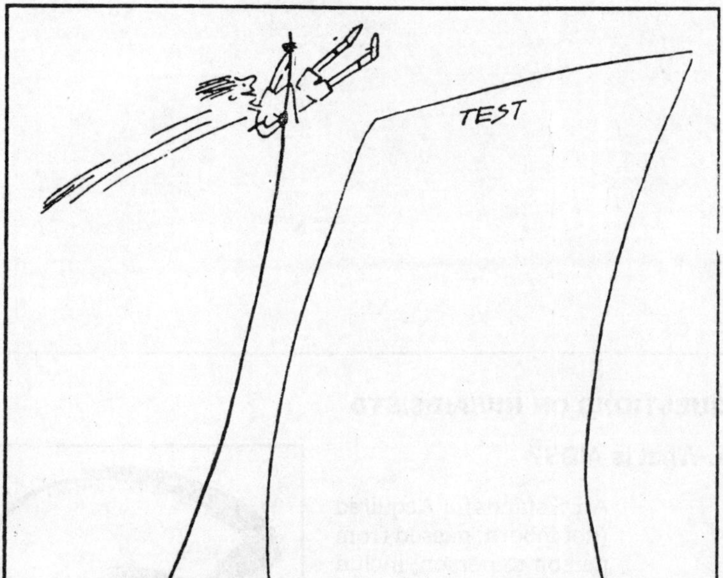

The best way to involve parents is...

[Provide here detailed guidance to teachers on how to involve parents, and the type of materials and activities that are envisaged for parents.]

Test items for student evaluation

Short tests are given for a number of reasons: to motivate students to learn the materials in the programme; to inform students of their progress; to produce a grade or mark; and to inform you of the progress of your students. The items in the following test have been selected to match the curriculum you have been teaching. It should be given to the students at [indicate here the timing: at the end of each unit, of each year...]

The correct answers should be discussed with the students after the test. Answers to the questions are provided for you so that you can mark and discuss the tests. [Add here the recommended test, with answers]

QUESTIONS ON HIV/AIDS/STD

1. What is AIDS?

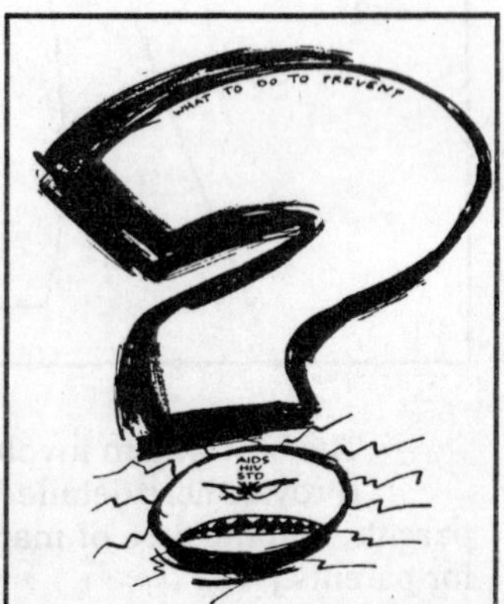

AIDS stands for Acquired (not inborn, passed from person to person, includ ing from mother to baby); Immune (relating to the body's immune system, which provides protection from disease-causing germs); Deficiency (lack of response by the immune system to germs); Syndrome (a number of

signs and symptoms indicating a particular disease or condition).
- AIDS is caused by a virus, called HIV (human immunodeficiency virus) which attacks and, over time, destroys the body's immune system.
- A person has AIDS when the virus has done enough damage to the immune system to allow infections and cancers to develop.
- These infections, cancers etc. make the person ill and lead to his/her death. At present, there is no vaccine or cure for AIDS.

2. What do we know about HIV?

- HIV, like other viruses, is very small, too small to be seen with an ordinary microscope. Viruses cause all sorts of diseases from flu (influenza) to herpes to some kinds of cancer.
- To reproduce, HIV must enter a body cell which in this case is an immune cell. By interfering with the cells that protect us against infection, HIV leaves the body poorly protected against the particular types of diseases which these cells normally deal with.
- Infections that develop because HIV has weakened the immune system are called "oppor tunistic infections". These include: respiratory infections e.g. tuberculosis; Pneumocystis carinii pneumonia; gastro-intestinal infections e.g. candidiasis in the mouth or diarrhoea, and brain infections e.g. toxoplasmosis or cryptococcal meningitis.
- Some people may also develop cancers, e.g. Kaposi sarcoma, a cancer which often cause red skin lesions.

3. What is an STD?

- STD stands for sexually transmitted disease or diseases. Many different STD have been identified. The most common STD include: gonorrhoea, chlamydia, syphilis, trichomonas genital warts, chancroid, genital herpes, hepatitis B and HIV infection.
- STD are caused by viruses, bacteria, and parasites. Viruses cause a number of STD, including genital warts, hepatitis B and genital herpes. Bacteria cause STD such as gonorrhoe, and syphilis. Scabies, trichomonas and pubic lice are parasite STD.
- Most STD can be cured.
- Certain STD infections, if not treated soon enough, can lead to long-lasting health problem in both males and

females, e.g. damage to the reproductive organs so that a woman is no longer able to have children cancer of the cervix, heart and brain damage, and possibly death.

- In many STD, the early symptoms are often difficult to recognize, and many people ignor them until more severe damage is done. This is especially true for women. This makes early diagnosis and treatment difficult.
- An abnormal discharge from the penis, anus or vagina; burning on urination; pain in the abdominal or groin area with a fever pain during sex; and rashes, blisters or sores on th genitals, are all possible symptoms of STD. If a person experiences any of the above symptoms, they should stop having sexual intercourse and go to a clinic or hospital for a check-up.

4. What are antibodies?

- The body's defense system (immune system) develops germ fighters, called antibodies to fight off and destroy various viruses and germs that invade the body.
- The presence of particular antibodies in a person's blood indicates that the person has been exposed to that infection. For example, when a blood test reveals that the antibodies to HIV are present in the blood, it means that the person is infected with HIV.

5. What is the "window" period?

- This is the time that the body takes to produce measurable amounts of antibodies after infection. For HIV, this period is usually 2-12 weeks; in rare instances it may be longer.
- This means that if an HIV antibody test is taken during the "window" period it will 10 negative since the blood test is looking for antibodies that have not yet developed. But the person is already HIV-infected and can transmit HIV to others.
- People taking the test are advised, if the result is negative, to return for a re-test in three months by which time if the person had been infected, the antibodies are almost certain, have developed (they should avoid risk behaviours during the 3 months).
- The most common test for HIV antibodies is called the ELISA test.

6. What does the asymptomatic period mean?

- The asymptomatic period is the period of time between infection and the beginning signs and symptoms related to AIDS.

- This varies from person to person for HIV/AIDS. It may be as short as 6 months or as long as 10 years or more.
- People usually have an asymptomatic period of several years in which they may have swollen Iymph nodes but no other complaints. Then, they may start to develop symptoms like oral thrush or night sweats. It may then still take years before they develop full-blown AIDS. The period between the development of full-blown AIDS and death may be as short as months or as long as 2 years or more.
- During the asymptomatic period there may be no evidence that the person is sick; however, HIV-related illnesses can occur regularly over many months or years before full-blown AIDS develops.
- During the asymptomatic period (as well as during the symptomatic period), the person infectious - that is, can pass HIV on to others.

7. What are the symptoms of AIDS?

- This question must be approached with caution in any specific case, since it is often diff cult to determine if the symptoms actually mean onset of AIDS or if they are simply symptoms of other conditions. People develop signs and symptoms of their HIV infection before they develop what has been defined as AIDS. AIDS is the final and most severe phase of HIV infection and leads to death. The obvious signs and symptoms are indications of an opportunistic disease such as tuberculosis or pneumonia. However, associated findings might include: recent, unexplained weight loss; fever for more than one month; diarrhoea for more than one month; genital oranal ulcers for more than one month; cough for more than one month; nerve complaints enlarged Iymph nodes; skin infections that are severe or recur.

8. Are there drugs and vaccines to treat AIDS?

- There are drugs that are effective against many of the infections associated with AIDS. These drugs are not a cure for AIDS but they can postpone symptoms or death.
- A few drugs have been able to inhibit the multiplication of HIV in infected persons. These, drugs do not eliminate the virus from the body but may be useful in prolonging life in patient who are infected with HIV.
- To date, there is some optimism over the development of a vaccine to protect against the disease. Part of the

difficulty is that there are many strains of HIV. Even within the same person the virus can change over time. Work is proceeding on this, but safe, effective vaccines are likely to take many years to develop.

9. How do you get HIV?

- HIVcan be found in body fluids like blood, semen, vaginal fluids, and breast milk.
- Any practice which allows the penetration of the virus from these fluids through the skin or mucous membranes and into the bloodstream of another person can cause HIV infection.
- The skin normally is a barrier to this type of penetration, but this barrier can be broken Breaks in the skin include such minor things as cuts, abrasions, sores and ulcers.

HIV is transmitted from person to person in 3 major ways:

i) When semen or vaginal fluid from an infected person comes in contact with the mucous lining (membranes) of the vagina, penis or rectum and the virus moves into the bloodstream.

ii) When the skin is penetrated by a needle, or other skin-piercing instruments (e.g. razor or tattooing instrument), and that instrument has blood on infrom an HIV-infected person. Sharing the same syringe and needle among injecting drug users is particularly risky for transmission. Any unsterile syringes and needles can transmit infection.

iii) HIV may also be transmitted from an infected mother to her baby, either through ths placenta before birth, during birth, or, in some cases, through breast milk after birth.

Note that:

- For medical reasons, it may be important for a person to receive a blood transfusion. If the blood donor is HIV-infected, there is a high chance that the virus would be transmitted through the blood. However, most countries now test donated blood for HIV and the chance of being infected in this way is very small.
- Deep wet kissing has a very low risk of transmitting HIV. However, there is a slight risk if there are cuts or abrasions in the mouth.
- Although the risk of infection is very low, it is advisable not to share toothbrushes.

10. How you don't get HIV?

- HIV is not transmitted by touch, coughing and sneezing, cutlery, glasses, cups and food, swimming pools, towels, toilet seats, pets, mosquitoes and other insects, baths or showers.
- Nurses, and other health service staff, who come in close contact with patients'body fluids, are trained to take precautions as part of the hospital routine.

11. How can one avoid infection?

- A person who does not engage in sexual intercourse and does not inject drugs (or who clean, sterile needles/ syringes for such injections) has almost no chance of contracting or other STD.
- Being married or not having sex before marriage cannot by themselves protect against HIV. Many people have believed this and have been infected by their partners. (This is especially true for many women for whom the only risk factor was having sex with their husband partner.)
- People who are mutually faithful (i.e. they only have sex with each other) are not at risk. HIV/STD by sexual means provided that both are HIV-negative at the start of their relationship that neither gets infected through blood (transfusion, injecting drugs with unclean needle/ syringe).
- People who use a condom correctly every time they have sex protect themselves from HIV/STD infection.
- Washing after sexual intercourse does not help to prevent HIV infection.

12. Do sexually transmitted diseases increase your chance of getting HIV?

- There is strong evidence that other sexually transmitted diseases put a person at a great risk of getting and transmitting HIV. This may occur because of sores and breaks in the skin or mucous membranes that often occur with STD.
- If you suspect you may have acquired or been exposed to an STD, you should seek medical advice.
- A person who has an STD should be aware that if they are having unprotected sexual intercourse, they are at an even higher risk of getting HIV.

13. What do "safe sex" and "protected sex" mean?

Because of the risk of HIV/AIDS, it is necessary to be very clear about the sexual practices which are known to carry a risk of HIV transmission and those which do not.

A)Safe sex activities(no risk)

- Practising the following activities will prevent a partner's blood, semen or vaginal secrations from getting into contact with your blood and thereby prevents transmission of HIV: masturbation, massage, rubbing, hugging, touching genitals.

B) Low-risk sex activitles

- Using a condom correctly and consistently during sexual intercourse, will reduce the risk of infection with HIV and other STD. Latex condoms have been demonstrated to be effective protection against HIV, STD, as well as pregnancy. Incorrect use of condoms reduces their effectiveness, e.g. they may break. Sexual intercourse with a condom is called "protected sex".
- While only a small number of people have contracted HIV through these means, the following activities are considered to carry some risk:
  - fellatio (mouth on penis without taking semen into the mouth);
  - cunnilingus (mouth on vagina);
  - anilingus (mouth on anus); and
  - deep wet kissing.

C) Unsafe sexual actzvities

- Practising the following activities is a definite risk:
  - anal sex (penis in rectum) without a condom;
  - vaginal sex (penis in vagina) without a condom;
  - any sex act that makes you bleed;
  - semen (or blood) taken into the mouth during oral-genital sex.

14. What is affection without sex (non-penetrative sex)?

There are many ways of showing affection and enjoying sexual pleasure like touching, masage, mutual masturbation. In many cultures, penetration is regarded as the only way of having sex. However, alternatives to penetrative sex are often enjoyed by women and men;

15. Do some people have a high likelihood of getting HIV?

Yes. It depends on a person's behaviour. Some behaviours/ activities carry a higher risk getting HIV than others. These include:

- Having many different sexual partners.
- Practising unsafe sexual activities, e.g. have sexual intercourse without a condom (see above, - Having sex when you have other sexually transmitted diseases.
- Sharing needles and syringes for injecting drug use.

Some situations which are beyond an individual's control can put them at risk. These include:

- Receiving injections with needles that are not cleaned or sterilized properly.
- Receiving blood transfusions with blood that has not been tested.

16. Are men and women equally vulnerable physiologically to HIV infection?

Women are slightly more vulnerable physiologically to HIV infection than men. The area of mucous membrane exposed during intercourse is much larger in the woman than in the man and the mucous membrane surface of the vagina (compared to the penis) can more easily be penetrated by virus. Very young women are more vulnerable than women in the 18-45 age group; their immature cervix and relatively low vaginal mucus production present less of a barrier to HIV. Women are becoming infected at younger ages than men. This is party because many young women marry or have sex with men older than themselves, who already had a number of partners, and partly because of their biological vulnerability.

17. Do you have to have many sexual partners to get infected with HIV/STD?

Even one contact with a person infected with HIV is enough to transmit the infection. However, the risk of getting infected with HIV increases with the number of sexual partners and the number of sexual acts. The presence of an STD (e.g. genital ulcers) in a sexual partner increases the risk of transmission of HIV.

18. Questions on transmission:

a) Is HIV spread by prostitutes and their clients?

Prostitutes and their clients, like any other people with many sexual partners, run the getting infected by their partners. They may then pass the infection to many others. If a prostitute insists on using a condom every time she or he has sex, the risk of infection and the partner will be sharply reduced. Many prostitutes have replaced penetrative sex with safer practices, further reducing the risk of infection. Unfortunately clients often refer wear condoms and the women are not in a position to insist.

b) If a woman is menstruating is there a greater risk of getting infected with HIV (for her partner and for herself)?

Menstrual blood from HIV-infected women does contain the virus. Infection would be dependent on whether the menstrual blood had contact with the sexual partner's bloodstreem. A woman who is menstruating is likely to be at a higher risk for HIV through sexual course.

c) Can you get infected by blood transfusion or by blood products?

Recommended standard practice for all transfusion services is to test and exclude from all blood and blood products that are "seropositive" i.e. contain antibodies to HIV. In most countries, efforts have been made to test all blood donations for HIV since 1985.

There is a very small chance that an occasional transfusion may contain the virus since an HIV-infected donor might have been in the "window" period (test negative) when giving blood.

You cannot get HIV from donating blood.

d) What happens to a baby born to a woman with HIV infection?

- The baby may be born infected with the virus. An infected mother can also pass the infection to her baby during breast-feeding after childbirth.
- About 20-40 percent of babies born to infected mothers will acquire the HIV virus. Some of those will develop AIDS during the first year of life. The majority of HIV-infected babies will not survive to their second birthday. However, some may survive up to 7 years or even longer.
- It serves little purpose to test babies born to HIV-infected mothers for HIV antibodies at birth. There are likely to be many false positive results because antibodies from the mother are still circulating in the baby's bloodstream. Only at 18 months or older, can an antibody test result be regarded as reliable.

e) Does breast-feeding transmit HIV?

Breast milk of an HIV-infected mother contains HIV which can be transmitted to the baby. However, because of the benefits of breast-feeding, the World Health Organization recommends that in situations where infectious disease and malnutrition are the main cause of infant deaths, and the infant mortality rate is high. mothers should breast-feed their babies, even if they are to be infected with HIV as the risk to the baby is less than the risks involved in artificial feeding.

19. Can needles, knives and other instruments transmit HIV?

Yes. Any instruments that cut the skin or puncture the skin can collect small amounts of blood that can be passed on if used again by another person without being sterilized. Avoiding, ear piercing, tatoo, acupuncture, blood-letting ceremonies or sharing razors unless you are absolutely sure the instruments being used are sterilized or boiled in water.

20. How is HIV transmitted with injection needles and syringes?

- Small amounts of blood remain in the needle and syringe after use. If someone else then use that needle and syringe, any blood left in the syringe or needle will be injected into their blood stream. If the first user was infected with HIV then the second person may now also be infected.
- Only a very small amount of blood is needed for transmission to occur. Sharing needles and syringes used for anything - medicines or heroin, cocaine, amphetamines (speed) and even water can spread HIV. It is not what is put into the syringe that transmits HIV, but the blood that remains in the needle and syringe.
- Some countries have needle and syringe exchange programmes (used needles and syringe: are exchanged for new ones) for injecting drug users. Those who cannot stop injecting drugs: can join these programmes to avoid HIV transmission.
- If people are not in a position to use a new needle and syringe, the equipment can be boiled or, if boiling is not possible, cleaned in the following way:
    - Rinse the syringe out with clean, cold water at least twice (not hot water). Squirt the used water down the drain.
    - Rinse the syringe out at least twice with fresh, household bleach, squirting the used bleach down the drain.
    - Rinse it out again, at least twice with clean, cold water to get rid of the bleach.
- Be extremely careful if you come across a needle or syringe in a park or street. Dispose of it safely without touching it with unprotected fingers.

21. Can you get HIV from contact sports where bleeding may occur?

- There is no evidence that any person participating in any sports activity has become infected with HIVfrom, or has transmitted HIV to, other participants.
- It is possible that transmission could occur if an HIV-infected athlete had a bleeding wound that came in contact with a cut in the skin or mucous membrane of another person. Even in such an unlikely event, however, the risk of transmission would be very low.
- Given this small possibility, it would be wise in contact sports where bleeding might occur (such as boxing) to follow these procedures:
  1) cleanse any cut with antiseptic and cover it well;
  2) if bleeding occurs, stop activity and wait until the bleeding has stopped and then cleanse and treat it with an antiseptic and cover it securely;
  3) latex gloves should always be worn when treating injured people.

22. Do mosquitoes or other insects spread HIV?

- The evidence clearly shows that HIV is not spread by mosquitoes and other insects. Fot example, bedbugs, lice and fleas in the households of people infected with HIV do not spread the virus to the other people living in these households.
- If mosquitoes were responsible for spreading HIV, then people of all ages would be infected. In fact, children before puberty are rarely infected, unless they were born to infected mothers or had a transfusion with infected blood.
- We know that HIV lives in some cells of the human body but that it does not live in the cells of insects. Therefore, mosquitoes and other insects are not a suitable home for HIV.
- HIV is not like the malaria parasite which lives very well in the mosquito and spreads to people when mosquitoes bite, because it is in the fluid that the mosquito injects.

23. When should one be tested for HIV?

Remember you need to be tested twice (see above).

There are advantages and disadvantages to being tested for HIV. It is a decision that should not be taken lightly and the implications of positive and negative outcomes should be faced in advance with the assistance of an HIV/AIDS counsellor.

A) Advantages of being tested:

If you are infected with HIV..

- You can receive early treatment and perhaps live longer.
- You can make decisions to take good care of yourself.
- You can develop a good emotional support system in the early stages of the disease.
- You can use new medications as they develop.
- Knowing that babies can be born with HIV, you can make decisions about whether you wish to get pregnant.
- You can inform your partner(s) that you have HIV.
- You can abstain from sex or use a condom during sex.
- You can avoid sharing items that come in contact with blood - razors, tweezers, needle and syringes.
- You will decide not to donate blood and other tissues.

If you are not infected, you will be relieved to know the result and will want to protect your self in the future.

B) Disadvantages of being tested:

- Learning that a person is infected with HIV can be very distressing. The degree of distres depends on how well the person is prepared for the news; how well the person is supported by family and friends; and, on the person's cultural and religious attitudes towards illness an death.
- A person who learns he/she is infected with HIV is likely to suffer from feelings of uncer tainty, fear, loss, grief, depression, denial and anxiety; the person must make a variety of adjustments.
- Partners and family are likely to suffer from the consequences of HIV testing as well as the infected person, whether they are also infected or not.
- A person who has tested positive for HIV may be discriminated against if the information is revealed.

C) Some important points about knowing one's HIV status:

- A person with HIV has the opportunity to make others more aware of the disease and to fight for tolerance and compassion for people with AIDS.
- However, they should think carefully about revealing their status since misunderstanding and discrimination do exist and may affect them and those they love.
- In many situations, families are the main source of care and support and the type of car and support for HIV-infected people may change depending on the stage of infection. Ths situation requires counselling for family members as well as for the person infected with HIV.

- All medical information, including HIV/AIDS status should be kept confidential.
- HIV-infected workers or students should not be discriminated against.
- HIV infection alone does not limit fitness to study or to work.
- HIV infection should not be a cause for termination of employment or schooling.
- At work or school, as elsewhere, HIV-infected people have a responsibility to behave ways that do not put others at risk of infection.
- Donating blood is a very irresponsible way to find out one's HIV status. If you want to be tested, consult your health care provider who will refer you to the appropriate counsellor.

D) HIV testing should always be preceded by counselling, which includes:

- Information about the test procedure and the many factors involved in testing, including emotional, social and medical consequences of a positive or negative result. Advantages and disadvantages of testing should be discussed and the decision to be tested should be made after careful consideration of all factors.

E) HIV test results should always be given with counselling which consists of a talk between the individual and the counsellor aimed at discussing the test result.

- If the result is negative, the counsellor will discuss the importance of prevention of HIV/STD in detail with the person in order to reduce his/her risks of infection in the future. The discussion will cover not only the methods available but the person's individual situation concerns and attitudes which may influence whether or not these methods are feasible and acceptable and will be used.
- If the result is positive, the counsellor will discuss with the person all the above in order that he/she avoid infecting his/her partner (or children), but also in order that he/she a reinfecting him or herself (which may hasten progression of the disease). In addition to this, the major task for the counsellor will be to offer compassion, support and practical advice, including referral to appropriate medical services, to the person to enable him/her to cope with stress and anxiety and to make personal decisions. Follow-up sessions to ensure can ingful, consistent and long-term support will be necessary.

F) gtesting and/or counselling is not available: One should discuss one's risk factors with someone knowledgeable and still make decis to use condoms or to abstain from sexual intercourse and avoid pregnancy.

24. How can one identify a person with HIV?

- It is not possible to know by physical appearance that a person has HIV, because the may remain in the body for many years without causing any symptoms or signs.
- Only a blood test taken after the "window" period can tell if a person nas HIV.

25. What happens if you live close to someone with AIDS?

Living near someone who has AIDS or who is infected with HIV will not give you HIV. You live quite safely in the same room with someone who has AIDS, provided that he or she ir your sexual partner and that you take precautions in handling body fluids (blood in particular.

Unit 1

Basic Knowledge on HIV/AIDS/STD

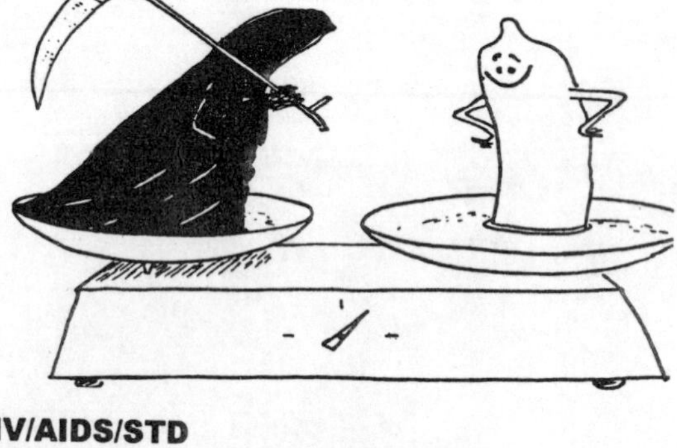

1.1. HIV/AIDS/STD
BASIC QUESTIONS AND ANSWERS

Purpose

To present basic information about HIV/AIDS/STD. Students need to be familiar with the terms that will be used in the rest of the programme. and understand why the programme is important to them. Teacher. will get a clear idea of the level of knowledge, attitudes and possibly some of the fears of their students.

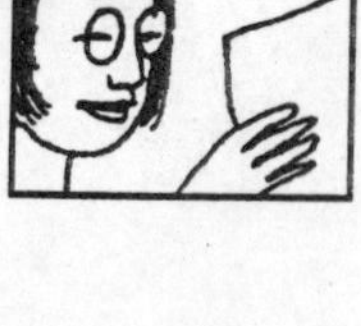

What the teacher does

This lesson could be developed in a number of ways:

1. Provide copies for each student, read the questions and the answers and provide additional explanation on new words.
2. Eight students ask one question each and the teacher responds to each question with the correct answer.
3. Leave the answers to each question blank and have the students provide the answers which they write into the spaces. This can be done individually, in groups or as a class activity.
4. The teacher could read each question and ask students for the answes.

Additional information

Since there may be additional questions from students when you do this activity, it would be important to read Questions on HIV/AIDS in this guide.

1.2. LOOKING INTO AIDS

Purpose

This test can be used as an activity by itself or as a review of Student Activity 1- Unit 1. It can provide a quick evaluation of how much the students already know about HIV/AIDS/STD.

What the teacher does

1. Read the "Why?" and "How?" to the students.
2. Decide how to give the test:
   a) Give each student a copy of the test.
   b) Read the questions to the students and have them write the answers. Read out meaning of their scores.
   c) Divide the class into two teams - choose one person from each team to give correct answer - one team gets the even questions and the other the odd ones. Time should be given for each team to come up with what they think the correct answer is Scores for each team are added and then the teacher and students can look at what the scores mean (see Students' Activities).
   d) Make sure that students correct any wrong answers in their books.

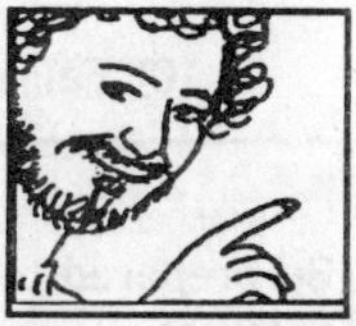

3. Provide the answers for the students which are given below:
   1) False: AIDS is a number of diseases that invade the body because HIV is Progressively destroying

the body's defenses (the immune system); AIDS caused by HIV.

2) False: It is HIV that damages the body's immune system.

3) True : It may be some time before a cure is developed. Some drugs can he prevent opportunistic infections.

4) True : Most people with AIDS will die within 6 months to 2 years after A has developed.

5) False: STD are sexually transmitted diseases - that is, diseases that are t mitted by sexual activity.

6) True: Many people have HIV or STD and do not know it. The sad part is th they can pass the infections on to someone else without knowing it. Some STD can cause severe damage if left untreated.

7) False: Since they are transmitted sexually or by using unclean needles, you can control these diseases by protecting yourself. These ways will be taken about later in the programme.

8) True : There are more than 20 STD; gonorrhoea is one of the more common STD among young people.

9) False : Women are slightly more vulnerable physiologically to HIV infection tha men. Women are becoming infected at younger ages than men. This is partly because many young women marry or have sex with men older than themselves, who have already had a number of partners, and partly because of their biological vulnerability.

10) False Anyone can get HIV/AIDS/STD.

Additional Information

Be prepared to answer additional questions when taking up the answers.

1.3. HIV/AIDS/STD

WHAT DO THEY MEAN?

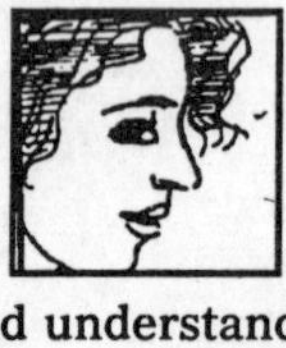

Purpose

Student should be familiar with basic terms and understand of these diseases in order to be prepared for the rest of the course.

What the teacher does

1. Decide how to teach this activity:

a) Each student receives a copy of the activity and follows the directions provided.

b) The teacher reads the story (A) and puts the definitions (B) on the blackboard. Students select the correct definitions from B and put them in the proper spot in C. The unfinished sentences are also put on the blackboard for students to complete.

2. Give the correct answers for each definition:

AIDS = Illnesses that occur...
HIV = A virus that...
STD = Diseases that are...
Gonorrhoea = A type of STD...

3. Provide additional infornation after each definition as below.

- AIDS is serious because:
  - there is no vaccine;
  - there is no cure;
  - anyone can get it (even young people);
  - it is almost certain that everyone who has AIDS, dies;
  - often they are young people who would otherwise have many years to live.

- After the definition for HIV, tell the students:
  - most people who have HIV have no signs of it;
  - unlike many other diseases, HIV does not get to us through air, water or food— you get it by sexual contact or sharing of unsterilized needles and syringes;
  - HIV cannot live outside the body for very long;
  - it is not carried by animals or insects.

- STD are serious because:
  - they can damage the reproductive organs;
  - they can cause infertility (inability to have children);
  - they can cause cancer, heart and brain damage, and possibly death.

- After the definition for STD, tell the students:
  - HIV/AIDS is an STD and so is gonorrhoea (give the local/slang name of gonorrhoea.
  - you should contact the health centre if you have pain in the genitals, or when urination. If you have ulcers in the genital area or an unusual discharge from the vagina penis.

    most STD can be cured.

4. Ask the students for their answers to the unfinished sentences.

   You might finish the class by asking them to respond to, "I learned from the class today that..."
   Be sure to give positive feedback to each appropriate answer that is volunteered by the students.

5. Have a cardboard box with "Dear teacher" on it where students can put their questions. Do not have them sign their questions. Read them and find answers for the next class.

Additional Information

The teacher may have to find answers to the students' questions. This should be done after class. You may need to find additional sources to answers all of the questions, like the professionals at the health centre or hospital. Do not be afraid to admit you could not find an answer to very difficult questions. Do not guess at answers—be sure the answer is correct.

1.4. HOW A PERSON GETS HIV

*(the virus that causes AIDS)

Purpose

To illustrate the three routes of transmission of HIV.

What the teacher does

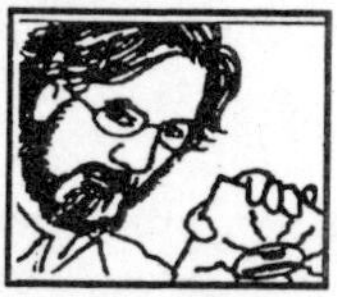

1. Decide how to teach this activity:
   a) A copy is given to each student and the teacher reads the information. The teacher asks questions and/or clarifies each route of transmission.
   b) If there is only one copy, the teacher reads the information and asks questions and/or clarifies each route of transmission.
2. Questions for clarification might include:

   - HIV spreads through sexual intercourse:
     a) What are other examples of STD?
        Chlamydia, gonorrhoea, genital warts, herpes.
     b) What fluids in the male reproductive system can contain HIV?
        Semen.
     c) What fluids in the female reproductive system can contain HIV?

Vaginal secretions, menstrual blood.

d) Where would the HIV in these fluids enter the person's body?
Through the mucous membranes that line the vagina, penis, anus/rectum.

- HIV is spread through infected blood:
  a) How could there be blood in needles or syringes?
  Blood left in needle or syringe from a previous injection into another person.
  b) What substances do people inject into their bodies?
  Drugs - heroin, cocaine, speed, steroids.
  c) Why would unsterilized tools contain blood, e.g. ear-piercing?
  Blood left in needle or on instrument from cutting or puncturing.

- HIV spreads from an infected mother to the unborn or newborn child:
  a) How would the babies get HIV?
  From mother's blood, during pregnancy or delivery; less commonly, througl breast milk.
  b) What could be done to prevent this from happening?
  A woman with HIV should seek advice and/or go for counselling as she may to avoid pregnancy.

What should be done by parent(s)

(if there is a parents' guide)

Either read the information sheet How a person gets HIV infection, or have child read the activity to the parents. The child could clarify questions about the information.

Additional preparation

Teachers should prepare for additional questions on transmission, particulalry if there are not follow-up activities on transmission.

1.5. YOU CAN'T GET AIDS BY.....

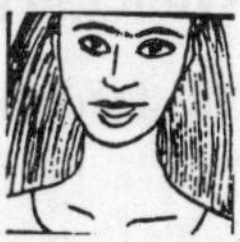

Purpose

As well as knowing how HIV is transmitted, it is important to know how it is not transmitted. This reduces irrational fears about the disease:

What the teacher does

1. Decide how to teach this activity:
   a) Hand out the activity sheet to the students and have them fill in the answers from the 12 pictures. Read with the students the information on the sheet.
   b) Put the students in small groups. Provide one activity sheet for each group. As a group they will fill in the answers from the 12 pictures.

2. Discuss the right answers. These are:

1) Shakii g hands	7) Mosquito or any other insect bit
2) Coughing, sneezing	8) Eating or drinking from same glass or plate as an HIV-infected person
3) Kissing on cheek	
4) Hugging	9) Swimming or bathing
5) Using a telephone or drinking from a fountain	10) Sharing a crowded bus
	11) Looking after pets or animals
6) Using a toilet	12) Wearing someone else's clothes

3. Ask the students if they can think of other activities that they think will not transmit HIV. Others might be: holding hands, giving blood, shar a towel, sharing combs, going to school with or touching someone with HIV.

What should be done by parent(s)

(if there is a parents' guide)

The parents can fill in the 12 answers from the pictures of the parents' guide. Parents and students can do the activity together.

1.6. WHAT DO YOU BELIEVE?

Purpose

To reinforce what has been learned about the ways in which HIV and cannot be transmitted.

What the teacher does

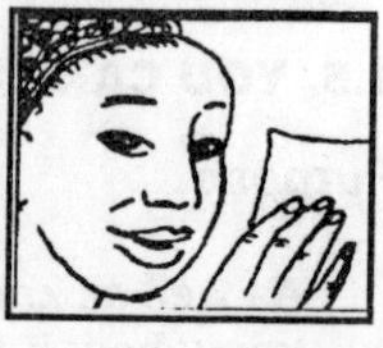

1. Decide how to teach this activity:
   a) Hand out this activity to the students and have them answer the question individually or with a partner.
   b) Form small groups and give five questions to each group. The group most correct answers is the winner.

c) Have two teams with captains for each team. They could be boys against girls if the class is co-educational. The captains give the answer after consulting with their team. One team does the even numbers, and the other the odd. Keep score blackboard.

d) Read the questions to the students and they answer true or false. Sheets for student are not needed in either method c) or d).

2. Give the students the correct answers. They are:

1) False — HIV cannot survive in air and so it is not spread by shaking hands.

2) True — In fact, the most common way for HIV to spread is through unprotected sexual intercourse with a partner who has HIV.

3) True — The AIDS virus can pass from the mother's blood to the baby's while it is developing in the mother or when the baby is being delivered.

4) False — Professionals who collect blood use new, clean needles to take blood from those who give blood. There is no danger in donating blood Donot give blood if you have HIV or have participated in risk behaviours.

5) False — Again, HIV does not live in air, nor is it transmitted through the skin (unless there are breaks in the skin).

6) False — There have been no known cases of HIV being transmitted by kissing. While it is true that the virus has been found in saliva, there are no reported cases of family members becoming infected by kissing, hugging and sharing eating utensils while caring for persons with AIDS. It might be possible if both partners had open sores in the mouth and have been "deep kissing".

7) True — If the blood of someone who has HIV is transmitted to another person who does not have HIV, there is a high risk of that person getting HIV. This happens mostly when people re-use unclean (not sterilized) injection needles and syringes and sharp instruments for tattooing, ear and nose piercing, circumcision, etc.

8) True — There are many cases of HIV being transmitted by drug users who share unsterilized injecting drug needles and syringes.

9) False — Although more men than women were reported with AIDS at the beginning of this disease, women are now being infected with HIV at the same rate

as men. Furthermore, women are biologically more vulnerable to HIV infection than men.

10) False — The AIDS virus does not live in air and cannot be passed from skin to skin (unless there are breaks in the skin).

11) False — HIV cannot be transmitted through swimming, bathing or drinking from water fountains.

12) False — Anyone can get HIV/AIDS.

13) False — A person can be infected with HIV, not be aware of it, and look perfectly healthy. During this time a person with HIV can pass it on to others.

14) False — If cutting or piercing instruments are not sterilized before re-use, the blood left on these instruments, when shared by others, can transmit HIV.

15) False — Re-used condoms may carry HIV, are more likely to break, and are more difficult to put on properly. Condoms should never be re-used.

16) True — Obviously, the more sexual partners you have, the more chance of being exposed to someone with HIV.

17) True — There have been no cases of transmission by these methods, even in people who care for people with AIDS.

18) False — Since these instruments may have blood left on them, it is possible that they could transmit HIV to another person. Although the risk of infection is extremely low, it is advisable not to share toothbrushes.

19) False — Although there are not many young people with AIDS, it should be remembered that HIV may be in the body for up to 10 years or more without signs or symptoms. Therefore, a person who is infected at age 15, might not get AIDS until the age of 25.

20) True — Since HIV is contained in blood, menstrual blood of an HIV-infected woman will contain HIV, that can be transmitted through any open sores or mucous membranes of her partner. More seriously a woman who is menstruating is likely to be at a higher risk for HIV through sexual intercourse.

What should be done by parent(s)?
(if there is a parents' guide)

This activity may be included in the parents' guide under "fun tests". Parents can do the test alone or with their child reading the questions and helping with the answers.

Additional preparation

Teachers should expect questions from students as they are giving the answers to the true-false questions. Be sure to review the information in this guide on questions young people ask.

1.7. WHAT WOULD YOU DO?

Purpose

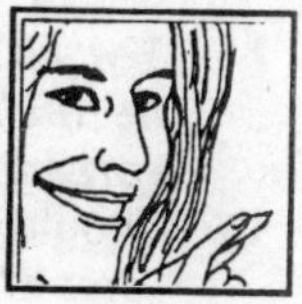

Stories about people's lifestyles, their risk of HIV and what they can do to prevent the spread are an effective way to describe risk situations to students in a realistic way.

What the teacher does

1. Decide how to teach this activity:
    a) Give each student an activity sheet and have them follow the instructions.
    b) Read each story to the students, ask them the questions under each story and put the risk continuum on the board. Ask various students to put the name of the character on the continuum where they think that person's risk is located (only one activity sheet is needed).
    c) Divide the class into three groups with a leader in each group. Give each leader one of the stories which they will read to the rest of the group. The group will then answer the questions and come to a consensus as to what risk the person in their story has for HIV/AIDS/STD. The leader will report on the answers (only three activity sheets needed or cut three stories out of one activity sheet).
2. Take up the answers with the students. Possible answers are provided below:

- ***Story 1***

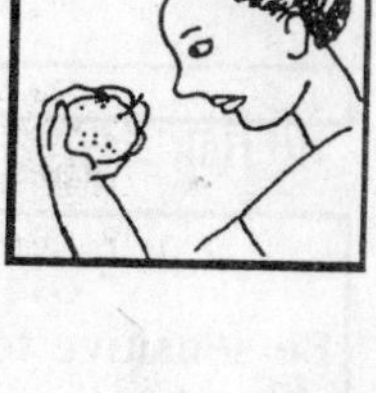

a) What could Natombie tell his mother about the spread of HIV?
He could say that there is no chance of him getting HIV/AIDS because it is only transmitted during unprotected sex and by dirty (bloody) needles, syringes or other instruments.

b) Does he need to quit his job? Why or why not?
No. In fact, if he did, it would be a pity because he has no chance of getting HIV/AIDS and he would lose valuable money.

c) Risk for HIV.

X

no risk low risk high risk

• ***Story 2***

a) Do you think he should continue going to school? Why or why not?
Yes, he should continue going to school since he feels well enough and becausc cannot spread HIV to other students.

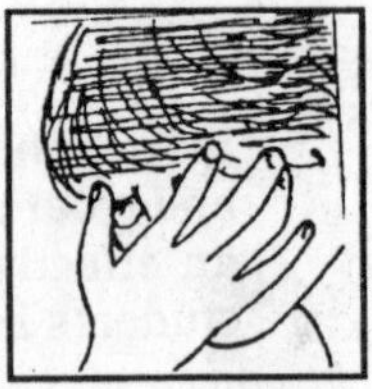

b) Should he tell anyone? Who? Why?
That is up to Haiwa, bu t probably a school official should know so that if he comes ill, the school will help him get proper care. He should get counselling to determine if he should tell others in the school.

c) How would you react if he told you?
You will get individual answers to this question but you should encourage student be supportive and help Haiwa whenever he needs help.

d) Risk for HIV.

X

no risk low risk high risk

• ***Story 3***

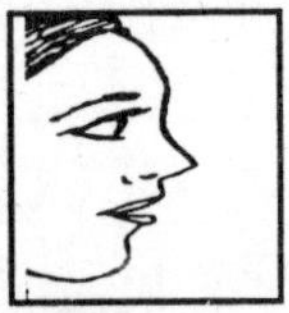

a) What should you tell Maria? Why?
You should tell her the truth - that is, that HIV is transmitted by sex and that if Rob has had sex with others (which you suspect he has) she had better: 1) not have sex with Roberto; 2) use a condom if she is going to have sex.

b) What risk would Maria have of getting HIV if she had sex with Roberto?
If they use a condom properly or if they use no protection.

with a condom no protection

X

no risk low risk high risk

Additional preparation

Be sensitive to the fact that some of your students may be in situations that are like the stories in this activity. You may want to remind the students that any questions or concerns are welcome after class in a private session with you.

1.8. WHAT IS YOUR RISK?

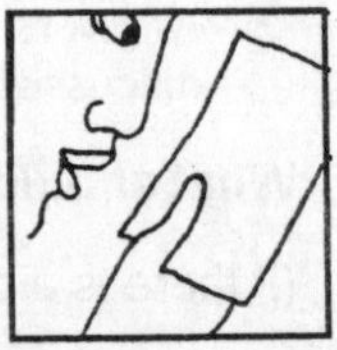

Purpose

Students will become more familiar with risk behaviours by classifying them as: No Risk; Low Risk; High Risk. They also need to evaluate their personal level of susceptibility based on their own risk behaviours.

What the teacher does

1. Decide how to teach this activity:
   a) Hand out an activity sheet to each student and have them follow the instructions (you may have to clarify the three categories of risk).
   b) Write each activity on the blackboard and have students discuss. Then you write NR, LR, HR next to each activity (no hand-out sheets are required). Place the continuum for "What is your risk" on the blackboard and let students visualize where they would put their "X". DO NOT HAVE THEM WRITE THEIR ANSWERS ON PAPER OR ON THE BLACKBOARD.
   c) Select two teams and two captains (peer leaders) - give one sheet to each - team 1 has questions 1 to 8 and team 2 has 9 to 16. Team captains read each activity and then take a vote - the winner is the team with the most correct answers. Have students draw the continuum for "What is your risk" on a sheet of paper and then decide where they are on the continuum. Do not let them write in their "X" - ask them to think about where they would put it.
2. Give the students the correct answers, and make sure that students place the correct answers in their sheets.
   1) NR Using toilets in a public washroom
   2) NR Touching or comforting someone living with AIDS
   3) HR Having sex without a condom
   4) LR Having oral sex (without semen in the mouth)
   5) NR Kissing (dry kissing)
   6) HR Having sex using the same condom more than once
   7) HR Sharing needles for injection drug use
   8) NR Swimming with an HIV-infected person
   9) HR Sharing needles for ear piercing or tattooing
   10) NR Abstaining from sexual intercourse
   11) NR Going to school with an HIV-infected person
   12) HR Cutting the skin with a knife used by others
   13) NR Being bitten by a mosquito
   14) NR Giving blood
   15) LR Having sex using a condom properly
   16) NR Eating food prepared by an HIV-infected person

3. Answers for "What is your risk?" are private and need not be discussed.

What should be done by parent(s)

(if there is a parents' guide)

Review the activity with their child (if each student has his/her own activity sheet).

1.9. ARE YOU AT RISK? (PART 1)

Purpose

Students learn to assess multiple risk behaviours by looking at a variety of activities. They then evaluate their personal level of susceptibility based on their own risk behaviours.

What the teacher does

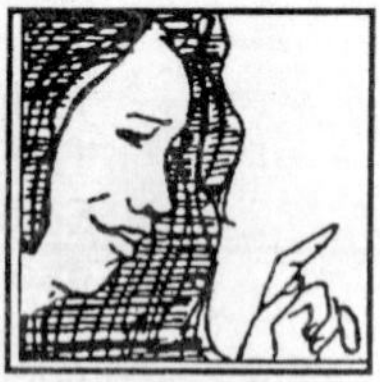

1. Divide the class into small groups (preferably 6 or 12 students in each group) and assign a leader to each group (to report back to the class and to direct and motivate the group).
2. Give each group a list of 6 behaviours/actions (you will have to repeat some lists if you have more than 6 groups).
3. Read the "How?" section to all of the students and explain to them how HIV can spread and the four risk levels (from the activity sheet).
4. Then assign them the task of deterrnining the risk level for each of their 6 behaviours/actions. Also assign the questions under "Teacher asks" to each group.
5. Write the 4 risk levels on the blackboard with lots of space for the students to write the numbers of the various behaviours/actions (see example below) or go over the 36 behaviours/actions having each group report their results (see next page).

No risk (NR)	Low risk (LR)	Sh risk (HR)	No agreement (?)
Behaviours/actions number	Behaviours/actions number	Behaviours/actions number	Behaviours/actions number

6. Review each behaviour/action when the students have finished writing on the board. Try to determine where the "No agreement" activities would go.

The answers are listed on the next page. There may be some questions about some of the behaviours/actions and if the doubt is reasonable allow that activity to be in more than one category. The high risk related to ejaculation into the mouth during oral sex and the low risk related to oral sex without semen in the mouth, might have to be discussed.

7. Have students place the correct risk factor for all 36 activities on their activity sheets (if they have been distributed to each student).

Group 1

NR 1. Body to body rubbing with clothes on.
HR 2. Sharing a razor to shave legs or face.
HR 3. Having sex with a condom - condom breaks.
NR 4. Back rub - massage.
NR 5. Riding on a bus with an HIV-infected person.
HR 6. Cutting the skin with a knife used by others.

Group 2

NR 1. Using toilets in a public washroom.
HR 2. Sharing needles for injection drug use.
NR 3. Being bitten by a mosquito.
NR 4. Dry kissing.
HR 5. Having vaginal sex without a condom.
HR 6. Cleaning up spilled HIV-infected blood without wearing gloves

Group3

HR 1. Having anal sex without a condom.
NR 2. Abstaining from sexual intercourse.
HR 3. Sharingneedlesforear-piercing.
NR 4. Shaking hands with an HIV-infected person.
LR 5. Having oral sex (without semen in the mouth).
NR 6. Swimming with an HIV-infected person.

Group 4

HR 1. Sharing needles for tattooing.
NR 2. Sharing clothes with someone who has HIV.
NR 3. Donating blood.
NR 4. Eating food prepared by an HIV-infected person.
HR 5. Having sex with a number of partners- no condom.
NR 6. Going to school with an HIV-infected person.

Group 5

NR1. Using public drinking fountains.

LR 2. Giving mouth-to-mouth resuscitation (if there are no sores in the mouth).
HR 3. Having unprotected sex with an STT)infected person.
NR 4. Playing sports with an HIV-infected person.
HR 5. Sharing a needle cleaned with water.
NR 6. Being close to an HIV-infected person who coughs or sneezes.

Group 6

HR 1. Being bitten by an HIV-infected person.
LR 2. Wet (deep) kissing.
LR 3. Having sex using a condom properly.
NR 4. Sharing a towel with an HIV-infected person.
NR 5. Touching or comforting someone living with AIDS.
HR 6. Having sex using the same condom more than once.

8. Discuss the answers to the questions under "Teacher asks".

Some young people become very afraid of HIV/AIDS.

a) Why do you think they are so afraid?	b) What could be done to prevent this fear of HIV/AIDS?
- their information is not very accurate; - the illness is serious and fatal; - they are unaware of how it can be transmitted; - they may have participated in risky behaviour	- get more reliable and accurate information; - talk to a medical expert; - get tested for HIV; - be aware of your risk behaviours.

1.9. ARE YOU AT RISK? (PART 2)

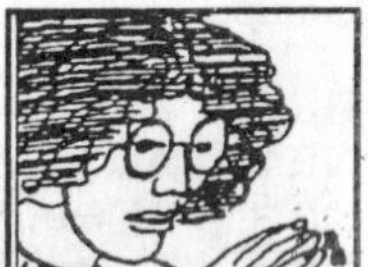

What the teacher does

1. Decide how to teach this activity.
   a) Give each student an activity sheet and have them follow the instructions.
   b) Divide the class into small groups and assign a peer leader ior each.
   c) Draw the diagram on the blackboard and read out the description of each person. Have the students discuss amongst themselves or in their group the unsafe behaviours for each person. Then have them rank the four people according to their behaviour, from safest to least safe (1-4). Only one activity sheet is needed if (c) is used.

- Person A: wet kissing and possibly touching genitals
- Person B: sex without a condom; boyfriend has used unsterilized needles and has had sex with a number of sexual partners without using a condom
- Person C: unsterilized needles for ear-piercing; sex with a condom
- Person D: no risk behaviours

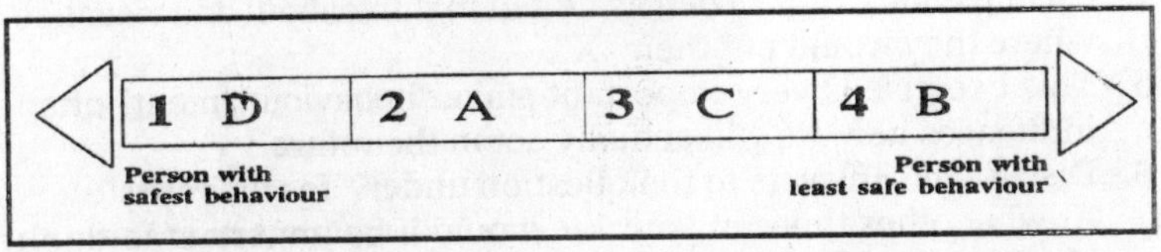

2. Discuss the answers to the question under "Teacher asks".

   What would the person in box 4 (B) have to do to reduce her chance of getting HIV/AIDS/STD?
   Answers will vary but they could include: not have sex; use a condom, ask her boyfriend to get tested; have non-penetrative sex.

Additional preparation

You must decide how you are going to form groups. It is better if the teacher does this rather than allowing students to form thier own groups. Groups should be no larger than 6. You should determine beforehand which peer leader will be with which group.

1.9. ARE YOU AT RISK? (PART 3)

What the teacher does

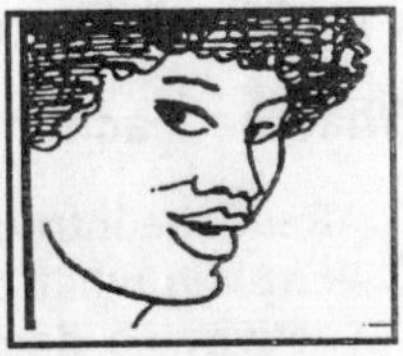

1. It is important for young people to think about and visualize their personal level of vulnerability (susceptibility). The continuum from left to right in part 3 allows students to determine their own risk.
2. Ask students to think about the risk activities they take - How many risk activities? How risky is each one? How often do they take them? Do they use protection? Do they use protection all the time?
3. After allowing them a few minutes to think about these questions, ask them to decide on a point on the continuum where they think they are. Notice that they cannot sit in the middle.

4. If the age level you are teaching is quite young, the risk level will probably be quite low for the majority of students. Therefore, it is important to have them think about and visualize where they might be five years from now. Questions you might ask: Do you think you might be in a relationship? Is there a chance it might involve sexual intercourse? Would you use condoms if it did? Consistently? Would you be assertive and insist on their use if your partner did not want to use them? Would you ever use injection drugs? Then ask them to think about and visualize where they would put their "X".
5. This exercise is very important since "behaviour intent" often influences how we will actually act in the future.
6. Discuss the answers to the question under "Teacher asks". At what other times in your life would it be important to think about your personal risk of getting HIV/STD? The best times to review your risk are when you decide to make changes in your sexual or drug behaviours.

What the peer leader(s) does (if used)

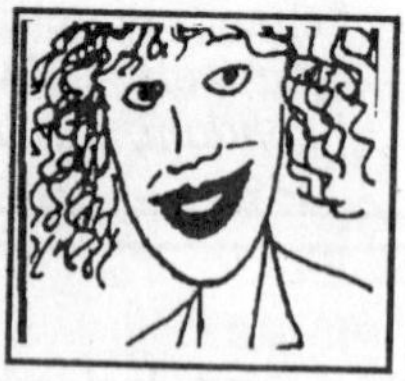

- They could be leaders in each of the small groups in part 1 and 2.
- They could be recorders and reporters for the small group decisions.
- They could hand out and collect materials.

1.10. PROTECT YOURSELF AGAINST AIDS

Purpose

It is essential that young people know how to protect themselves from HIV/STD. This activity provides information on, and encourages: discussion of safer choices of behaviour in relation to sexual intercource; unsterilized needles; cutting of the skin.

What the teacher does

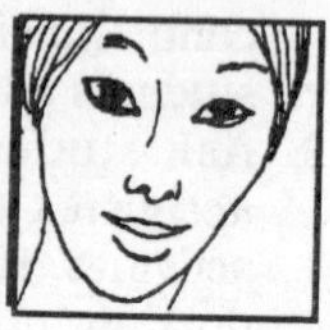

1. Read the introduction to the activity.
2. Explain what the students have to do in the activity, i.e. decide on safer choices for 1, 2 and 3.
3. Provide the answers for the students:
   a) Sexual intercourse
      - delay sexual intercourse;
      - be faithful to a partner who is free of HIV and is faithful to you;
      - love carefully

- use a condom correctly.

b) Unsterilized/shared needles and syringes (or other injecting equipments).
   - always go to a doctor, clinic or hospital for injections; they use sterilized needles
   - use new or clean (sterilized, boiled) needles if you must use an injection needle and syringe;
   - clean the needle and syringe with bleach if new ones cannot be obtained. Needles and syringes made of glass can also be boiled (see section 7 of this manual).
   - stop using injection drugs.

c) Avoid unsafe blood contact
   - refuse traditional cutting of the skin unless you can bring your own clean razor;
   - make sure sterilized tools are always used for tattooing, ear piercing, circumcisions;
   - it is advisable not to share toothbrushes; there is a very slight risk of blood to blood contact.

Additional preparation

Teachers should know about using condoms and how to clean a dirty injection needle (included in this guide). You may need to discuss condom use in terms of future use, particulalry if your community is opposed to discussing or advising condom use with young people.

1.11. DEAR DOCTOR SUE

Purpose

The medical profession is viewed as a reliable source of information about HIV/AIDS/STD. Dear Doctor letters allow students the opportunity of role-playing a health professional and comparing their advice to that of an actual doctor.

What the teacher does

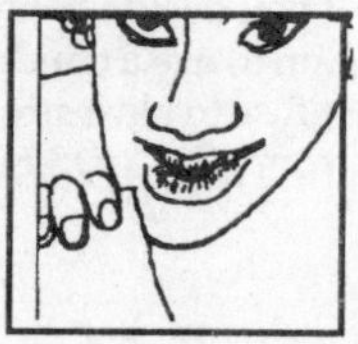

1. Decide how to teach this activity
   a) Provide a sheet for each student in the class and have them write one or more of the letters individually.
   b) Divide students into a number of small groups and give each group one letter. Have each group do one or more of the letters.
   c) Read the letter to the students and have individuals, pairs or small groups talk about or write a response. The

"Doctor's bag" would have to be written on the black board. (You only need one activity sheet for this method.)

2. Read the "Why?" and "How?" part of this activity to the students. Explain that they will write responses to the three letters as though they were doctors (individuals, pairs or small groups). Remind the students that the topic is protection from HIV/STD.
3. Explain that their letters will be compared to letters that have actually been reviewed by doctors who are experts in HIV/AIDS/STD. Tell them that young people often give good information and that their letters can be very useful to others.
4. Explain that they have a "Doctor's bag" of ideas to help them.
5. Ask a number of students or groups to read their first letter. Then read the actual doctor's letter (see next page) and ask the students to compare answers. Do the same thing for the second and third letters.

Additional preparation

You may think of additional things that could be put in the "Doctor's bag that are more applicable to your community.

Actual letters from doctors

Dear Norah,

You have made an important first step in writing this letter. I hope I can help you. Let me first say that you should do what you think is best for you and you shouldn 't let someone else make that decision for you. It seems to me that your feeling of not wanting to have sex at this time in your life is a good idea. Often if you can delay having sex for a few years you will make better decisions and be more responsible about avoiding unwanted pregnancy and HIV/AIDS/STD. There are many ways of showing affection to your boyfriend without actually having sexual intercourse. Suggest to him that everyone is not doing "it" and there are other ways of showing each other love. Tell him about some of these and ask him to tell you about any he knows. You may have to be assertive with your boyfriend to get him to understand. Remember that no boy is worth having who doesn't listen to you or respect your feelings.

If you decide to have sex with your boyfriend, it is absolutely necessary for him to use a condom properly. If he doesn't wish to or won't buy them, then refuse to have sex. Remember, condoms are the only way to protect yourself from HIV/AIDS/STD.

Yours sincerely, Doctor Sue

Dear John,

Let me say first that your compassion and worry for your brother is very kind. I think Abine has a true brother in you. Abine has at least three problems. First, in using a knife with someone else's blood on it, he has possibly exposed himself to HIV. Second, since he thinks he has an STD, I assume he has had sex with someone. If he has caught an STD, he is at higher risk for HIV and since he didn't use protection while having sex, he could pass the STD and possibly HIV to others. Third, the fact that he doesn't get much sleep, has a poor diet and smokes means that his body's defense against germs is lower. I feel that you should immediately talk to Abine about visiting a doctor, clinic or hospital. Tell him you will make the appointment and will go with him. I hope this information will help you.

Yours sincerely, Doctor Sue

Dear Allana,

I think you must be very worried and I hope I can help you. Sometimes worry stops people from taking action to do something about their situation. Often worries are needless if that there is no problem. You must go to a doctor, clinic or hospital for a check-up. If you find this difficult, find a friend or adult to go with you. A friend or adult to talk to is very important. If you have a problem, you will be given help and advice. If you don't have a problem and there is a good chance you don't, you must do one of the following. You should perhaps delay having sex until you are ready. If you continue having sex you should consider reducing the number of sexual partners and insist on the proper use of a condom which will protect you from pregnancy and HIV/AIDS/STD. Good luck.

Yours sincerely, Doctor Sue

1.12. WHICH IS SAFER?

Purpose

Students need to know ways of protecting themselves but they also need to know that some ways are better than others.

What the teacher does

1. Decide how to teach this activity
   a) Hand out a copy of the activity sheet and instruct the students to do the activity individually, in pairs or in small groups.
   b) Write the different activities on the blackboard and discuss the answers with the class as a whole or have the students do it on paper at their desks (only one sheet needed).

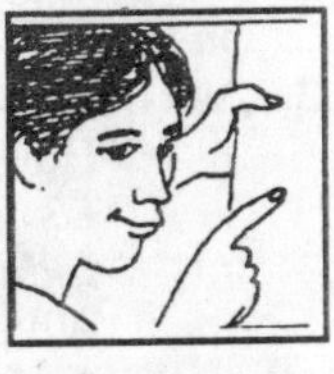

c) Put the students in small groups and hand out one sheet to each group.

2. Read and explain each of the "Protection against HIV/STD" methods.
3. Explain the "How?" of this activity, perhaps giving an example on the blackboard.
4. Have the students decide on the proper ranking and any problems with these methods of protection.
5. Discuss the correct ranking and problems. These are listed below.

SAFEST

Method	Problem(s)
Abstinence	this is difficult for a person's whole life
Kissing,etc.:	becomes risky only if blood, vaginal secretions, semen are exchanged
Condom:	if not used properly, it may break
One partner:	your partner may be already infected and not know it; partner must be 100% faithful
History:	many lie to have sex, are unwilling to tell everything
Few partners:	sex with one infected partner is enough to become infected with HIV
Get tested:	both partners need to be tested; you can get infected (e.g. by not being faithful) after being tested; one test is not enough

LEAST SAFE

1.13. WHAT HAPPENS WITH HIV INFECTION?

Purpose Students should be familiar with: the window period; time from infection to AIDS; time from AIDS to death; signs and symptoms of HIV/AIDS.

What the teacher does

1. Provide a copy of this information sheet for each student, or put the information on the blackboard.
2. Ask the students the following questions:
   - How long is the "window" period? *Usually 2-12 weeks but in some individuals it may be longer.*
   - What is not present in the blood during this period? *Antibodies to fight HIV, the AIDS virus.*

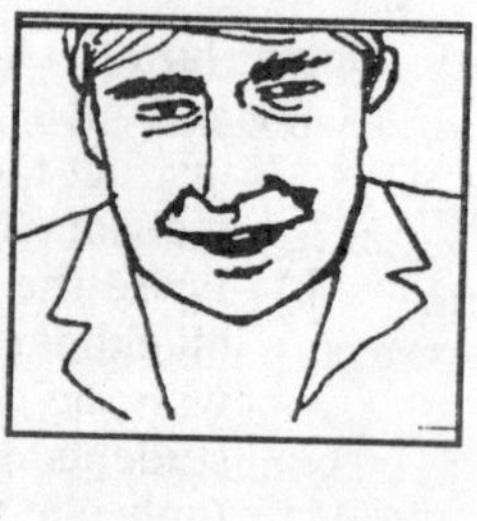

- What would happen if you got tested during this period?
  You would test negative because the test is looking for antibodies to HIV, which have not formed yet; the end of the "window" period is when there are enough antibodies to HIV in the blood that the test is able to detect them.
- Are people infectious (able to pass HIV on to others) during the "window" period?
  During the "window" period, people may be very infectious, and can pass HIV on to others.
- How could they pass these infections on to others?
  Through blood, semen or vaginal fluids or from mother to baby.
- What symptoms is a person likely to have during the first few weeks after infection with HIV?
  Immediately following infection there may be flu-like symptoms, with fever and swollen glands. Some people have fever, swollen glands, sore throat, skin rash or other symptoms in the days or weeks that follow infection.
- What is the possible length of time from infection to the beginning of AIDS?
  It varies a lot from person to person - it can be as short as six months or as long as 10 years or more.
- What are the signs and symptoms during this period of time?
  People usually have an asymptomatic period of several years in which they may have swollen lymph nodes but no other complaints. Then, they may start to develop symptoms like oral thrush or night sweats. It may then still take years before they develop full-blown AIDS.
- Is the person infectious during this period?
  Yes, HIV can be passed to others.
- How long is a person likely to live once they get AIDS?
  It varies; approximately six months to two years or more.
- What are the symptoms of AIDS?
  Major weight loss; persistent cough; fever or diarrhoea; and many others. They vary a great deal from person to person.
- Are people with AIDS infectious?
  Yes; any time after someone has been infected with HIV, whether they have symptoms or not, they can pass HIV on to others.
- What are ways in which the infection cannot be passed on?
  Hugging, glasses and dishes, touching, toilets, insects, etc.

What should be done by parent(s)

(if the Parents' Guide is used)

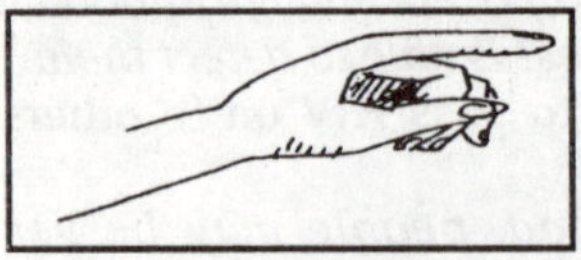

This activity is included in the Parents' Guide under "Information sheets". Students can explain the various parts of the activity to their parents.

Additional preparation

- Teachers should be knowledgeabl e about the progression from infection with HIV to AIDS. The above questions and answers will help and should be reviewed before doing the activity with students.
- This activity may cause some anxiety in students. Teachers should be prepared to offer sources of help to students who may approach them with concerns.

1.14. HOW DO YOU KNOW IF YOU HAVE HIV/AIDS?

Purpose

It is important for students to know that a person with HIV:

- May have no signs or symptoms for a long time.
- Can infect others during this time.
- Gradually gets sicker and sicker and eventually dies.

What the teacher does

1. Decide how to teach this activity.
    a) Provide each student with an activity sheet and have them do the activity ind vidually or in pairs, following the instructions on the sheet.
    b) Read the three stories to the students and ask the questions under each sto: (only one sheet is needed for the whole class).
    c) Divide the class into small groups each of which reads one story and answe questions (only one sheet for each group is needed).

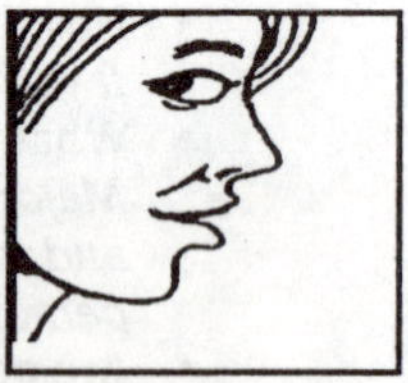

2. Review the information from activity 13 - unit 1.
3. Take up the questions under each story. The answers are provided below:

• ***Story 1***

Questions

1) How did Roberto become infected?
2) How did Carmencita become infected?
3) Why does Carmencita have no symptoms?
4) How long might it be before she gets AIDS ?
5) What should Carmencita do now?

Answers

1) Used unsterilized needles to inject cocaine.
2) By having unprotected sexual intercourse.
3) People with HIV may not have symptoms for many years.
4) It can be as long as 10 or more years, or as short as 6 months.
5) She should get counselling for support, including advice on lifestyle and sexual behaviour.

• ***Story 2***

Questions

1) How did Jose become infected?
2) Why does he have these symptoms?
3) Can he spread HIV to others? How?
4) What is likely to happen next?

Answers

1) Sex with no condoms; multiple partners.
2) They often occur as the earliest symptoms
3) Yes. By having unprotected sexual intercourse by sharing unclean needles and syringes.
4) He will probably get sicker and sicker.

• ***Story 3***

Questions

1) Why would you suspect that Georginia has AIDS?
2) What should she do to find out if she is infected with HIV?
3) About what age was it possible that Georginia got the HIV infection?

4) If she was infected at that age, how long has she been infectious (able to spread HIV)?
5) What symptoms does Georginia have?
6) What is likely to happen next?

Answers

1) She has many symptoms of AIDS.
2) Get tested, see a doctor or nurse.
3) From approximately 14 years onwards.
4) Up to 11 years.
5) Fever, sweating, swollen glands, cough, sore throat, stomach problems, weight loss.
6) She will probably die.

Additional preparation

- Be sure toreview the answers to the quesitions (above).
- Again, this activity may create some anxiety in students. Teachers should be prepared to listen and provide sources of help if needed.

1.15. TESTING FOR HIV

Purpose

Basic information about testing may be needed by some students.

What the teacher does

1. Decide how to teach this activity:
   a) Have a peer leader or student read the questions by Marie. The teacher respond as Dr. Matago.
   b) The teacher reads both the questions and answers or attempts to obtain answer from the students.
   c) Two students or peer leaders read the questions and the answers.

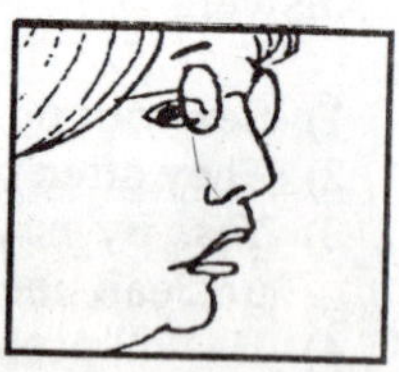

2. A pause should occur after each question and answer to allow student to ask additional questions.
3. The follow-up test (activity 16) should be given to students to test thei: attention and understanding (if there is enough time).

Additional preparation

- It is important that you read the section When Should One Be Tested for HIV?
- Teachers should be prepared to answer questions about testing facilities and practices in their local area, and what to do if counselling and/or testing are not available.

1.16. TEST: WHAT YOU KNOW...ABOUT TESTING

Purpose

This activity will help students recall information and understand concepts about testing.

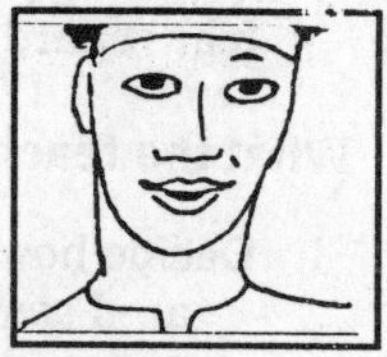

What the teacher does

1. Decide how to teach this activity.
   a) Provide each student with an activity sheet and have them do the test individually or in small groups.
   b) Put column B on the blackboard and read each statement from column A. Have students select the correct response (only one sheet needed).
   c) Place column A and B on the blackboard and have students do the activity individually or in small groups (only one sheet needed).

Note: For any of the above methods, it is possible to divide the class into two or more teams and have them compete.

2. Discuss the answers (provided below).

	Answers
The number of times you need to be tested in three months is:	G- twice
The test is accurate to:	I - 99%
It is important to take the test so that you can:	J - tell your partners/F - not infect others
It is also important to take the test so that you will:	F - not infect others/J - tell your partners
The most common test for HIV is called:	D - ' ELISA"
When no one else is told about the test that means that it is:	H - confidentlal
If you have HIV, you will be given:	A - advice and help
You can get tested at:	C - health centre or hospital
The test for HIV looks for:	E- antibodies
To get the results you probably have to:	B - come back later

Additional preparation

Be sure to go over the answers before doing the test.

1.17. AIDS HELP WHO? WHERE?

Purpose

Information on help sources for HIV/AIDS/STD is essential for young people. Some students may develop AFRAIDS (acute fear regarding AIDS) and may need help and counselling.

What the teacher does

1. Decide how to teach this activity.
   a) Pass out the activity sheet to each student and have them work individually, in pairs or in small groups to provide the answers to the four situations.
   b) Read each situation to the students and ask them the questions. If they don' t know the answers, provide the information for them.

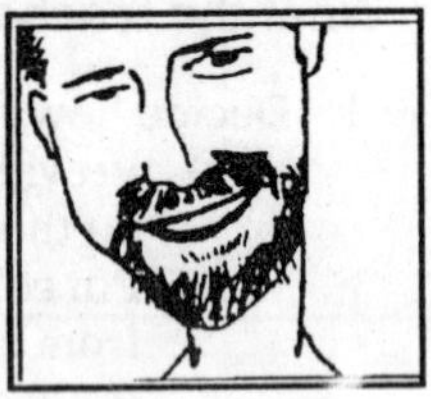

Note: In some cases, the answers for all four situations will be the same.

Additional preparation

Be sure to find sources of help if they are not available in your community (i.e. the nearest source of help; informed people in the community).

2. Be sure, before doing this activity, to identify the sources of help in your own community.

1.18. YOU BE THE DOCTOR

Purpose

Information about drug use and abuse and its relationship to HIV/AIDS is important. The following topics are discussed:

- Drug use and impairment of judgement
- Abstaining from injection of drugs
- Clean needle use for injection drugs
- Method of sterilizing unclean needles

What the teacher does

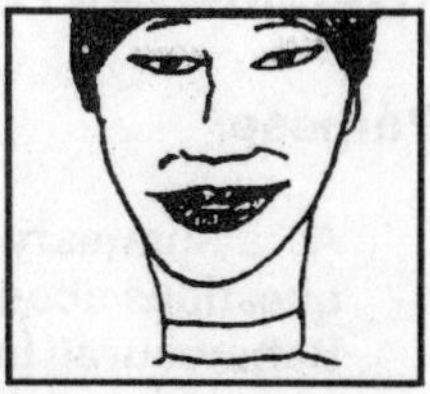

1. Decide how to teach this activity.
   a) Provide each student with an activity sheet and have them provide advice for one or more of the four situations individually, in pairs or in small groups.
   b) Read each situatlon and have students provide advice (and why) from the doctor's bag which is written on the blackboard (only one activity sheet is needed).
   c) Divide the class into small groups and give each group one or more situations for which to provide advice (only one activity sheet is needed for each group).
2. Have students read out their advice for each situation and discuss. Exarnples of appropriate advice are provided below:

• ***Situation 1***

a) Advice: Don't use drugs and alcohol—they slow your judgement.
b) Why? You might make decisions that cause you to get pregnant or HIV/STD.

• ***Situation 2***

a) Advice: Get clean (new) needles and syringes if you must use drugs.
b) Why? Used needles and syringes will have small amounts of blood left in them, which may contain HIV.

• ***Situation 3***

a) Advice: Never use injection drugs.
b) Why? They can be damaging to your health and there is a possibility of getting HIV/STD.

• ***Situation 4***

a) Advice: Clean needles with bleach and water if you must use drugs.
b) Why? There will be blood on the dirty nearile that mav contain HIV.

3. Students should be aware of how to clean needles and syringes. The procedure for this is found in the "questions" section of this guide.

1.19. ARE YOU A RESPONSIBLE PERSON?

Purpose

As a summary to this unit, students are asked a number of questions about their behaviour and their behavioural intent. Behavioural intent indications may be good motivators to produce desired behaviour in the future.

What the teacher does

1. Decide how to teach this activity.
   a) Provide an activity sheet for each student and have them do the activity individually.
   b) Read out each question and have students write 3 for *yes (agree)*; I for uncertain and 0 for no *(disagree)*. Only one activity sheet needed.
   c) Write the questions on the board and have students do the activity individually (only one activity sheet needed).

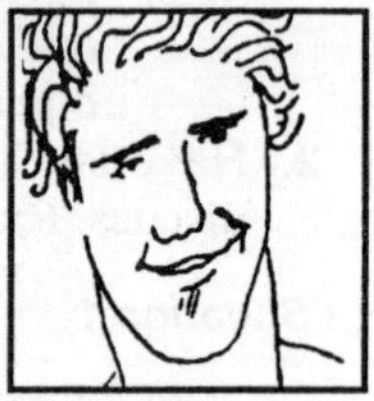

2. Students should total their score and refer to their "Responsibility score".

		Responsibility score	
Yes	=3 points	33-36 points	Very responsible
Uncertain	=1 point	30-33 points	Responsible
No	= 0 point	27-29 points	Somewhat responsible
		26-26 points	Not very responsible
		0-24 points	You are taking risks Maybe you should think again.

Additional preparation

Introduce this activity by telling the students that this activity is private (confidential) and scores will not be seen by the teacher or other students (unless revealed by the student).

Unit 2

Responsible Behaviour: Delaying Sex

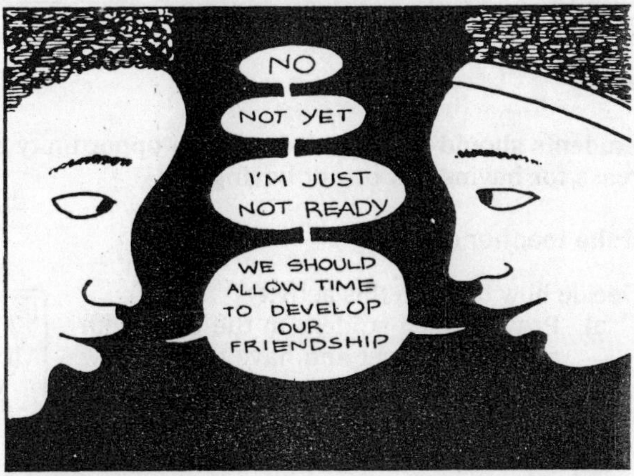
NO
NOT YET
I'M JUST NOT READY
WE SHOULD ALLOW TIME TO DEVELOP OUR FRIENDSHIP

2.1. REASONS TO SAY NO

Purpose

It is important for students to know a variety of reasons for delaying sex.

What the teacher does

1. Decide how to teach this activity.
   a) Provide each student with an activity sheet so that everyone can do the activity.
   b) Write the activity on the blackboard and have students do it on a plain piece of paper (only one activity sheet needed).

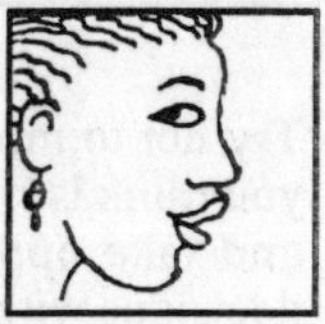

2. Have students choose the four reasons they think young people usually have for delaying sexual intercourse.
3. Take a poll, by show of hands and discuss with the students the top three or four reasons for delaying sex. You might want to ask:
   a) W'ıy they chose each reason as the top three or four.
   b) Do they think their reasons rnight change as they get older? How?
   c) Which of the four would be the best or most important reason (take another vote) and why?

Additional preparation

Depending on your community, there may be other reasons for delaying sex than those listed in this activity. If so, you should include these in the list.

2.2. TO DELAY OR NOT TO DELAY

Purpose

Students should be provided with an opportunity to explore reaso for having sex or not having sex.

What the teacher does

1. Decide how to teach this activity.
   a) Provide each student in the class with an activity sheet and have them follow th~ instructions individually, in pairs or in small groups.
   b) Read the story of Stoli and Yarmella and ask students to evaluate, as you rea~ them, each reason for saying "yes" as 0 = poor reason, or 1 = good reason. Do th same thing for reasons for Stoli and reasons for Yarmella to say "no". (Only on activity sheet needed.)

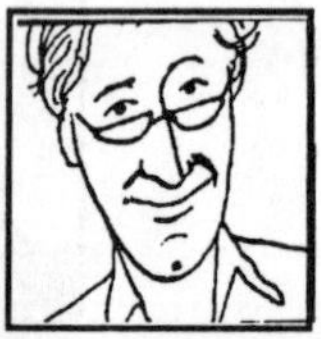

2. Encourage discussion by asking the questions in "Teacher asks". Yo will probably have to poll the class to determine the answers to some o these questions. Answers will vary from person to person and class to class.

Additional preparation

Try not to moralize or push students into making a decision that you think is right or proper. This will often cause students to rebel and take opposite point of view. They should make their own decisions without pressure.

2.3. "LINES" AND MORE "LINES"

Purpose

Students need practice in responding to typical arguments that are used to pressure individuals to have sex.

What the teacher does

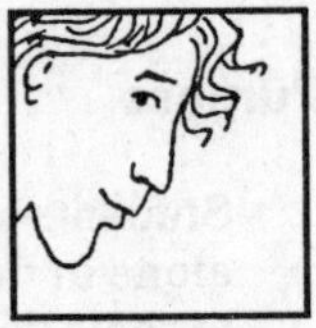

Notice that for every reason for not having sex (in activity 1 and 2 - unit 2), lines have been invented to persuade someone to forget their reasons a
d say "yes" to sex.

1. Decide how to teach this activity.
   a) Distribute an activity sheet to each student to complete individually, in pairs or in small groups. You may decide to divide the students into two groups so that each group only does 5 lines.
   b) Draw 10 question and answer "bubbles" on the board. Discuss an answer to each one and have a student place the best response in the "bubble" (only one activity sheet needed). You would need to put the list of "possible responses" on the blackboard.
   c) Divide the class into small groups - assign 5 lines to a group and have them decide on the best response (only one activity sheet per group is needed).
2. Add to the list of possible responses by asking students to suggest "lines" that they have heard.
3. Place the best response for each "line" in the appropriate bubble. There may be more than one good response.
4. Discuss or role-play.
   a) The best way to make your response - verbally and non-verbally?
   b) Try role-playing 5 or 6 responses by having two people say the "lines" and responses. Talk about the verbal and non-verbal actions of the role-players.

What the peer leader(s) does?

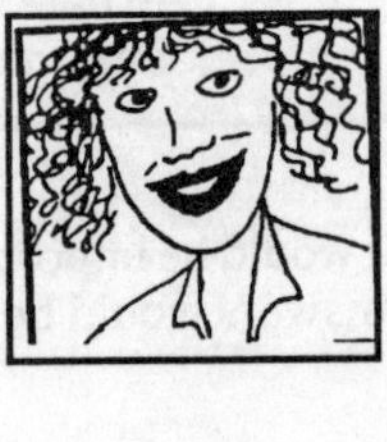

- Be in charge of a small group.
- Draw the "bubbles" on the blackboard (if that method is used).
- Role-play the lines and responses to the lines.

Additional preparation

Teachers should decide on appropriate responses for each line before doing this activity with students.

2.4. GUIDELINES: HELP TO DELAY SEX

Purpose

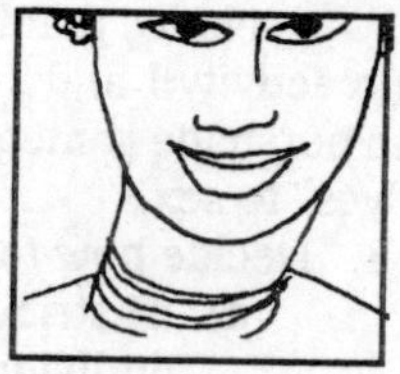

Students need to know that they are not alone in delaying sex. They also need help in their decision to delay sex.

What the teacher does

1. Decide how to teach this activity.
   a) Provide an activity sheet for each student and have them do the activity individually.
   b) Read each "Help for delaying sex" and have students put an "E" for easy to do and "D" for difficult to do (only one activity sheet needed).
   c) Write the activity on the blackboard and have students complete it individually (only one activity sheet needed).

2. Discuss the following:
   a) Which ones did the students find difficult? Why were they difficult? (Answers will differ from student to student.)
   b) Which of the guidelines would be best to avoid unwanted sex with a friend 9 (Answers could include many of the guidelines.)
   c) Which guidelines would be most useful for selecting who to go out with? (Answers will differ from student to student.)
   d) Which guidelines would be most helpful for a first date? (Answers will vary but the first six would be important.)
   e) Which guidelines would you use if you really didn't want to date at this time in your life? (Answers 1, 7, 8 would be important.)

Additional preparation

It would be important to review the above questions to decide what answers would be acceptable for each question.

2.5. WHAT TO DO?

Purpose

Students need to practise using the guidelines for delaying sex in life situations.

What the teacher does

1. Decide on a method for doing this activity.
   a) Provide an activity sheet for each student and have them work individualy pairs or in small groups.
   b) Write the list "Help for delaying sex" on the blackboard and then read aloud situation. Ask students to select the 3 best ways (from the list on the board) of he the person in each situation (only one activity sheet needed).
   c) Divide students into small groups and provide one sheet for each group (only one sheet per group needed).

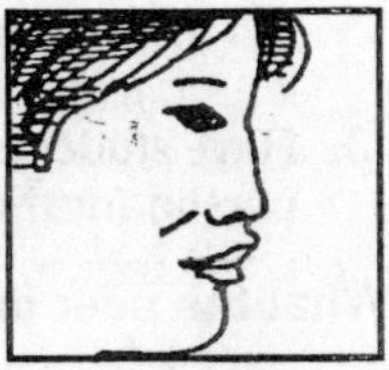

Note- If you need more tlme for this activity you might have one third of the class or groups do one situation each.

2. Provide the answers for each situation. These may vary from grot group and student to student and are only suggested answers.

• Situation 1

Help for Jeline

1) Decide how far you want to "go" (your sexual limits) before being in a pre situation.
2) Be honest from the beginning, by saying you do not want to have sex.
3) Decide your alcohol limits before being in a pressure situation.

• Situation 2

Help for Romain

1) Avoid going to someone's room (or house) when there is no one else there.
2) Be honest from the beginning by saying you do not want to have sex.

3) Pay attention to your feelings; when a situation becomes uncomfortable, leave.

• Situation 3

Help for Nadino

1) Do not accept presents and money from people whom you do not know very well.
2) Avoid secluded places where you could not get help.
3) Be honest from the beginning, by saying you do not want to have sex.

3. Have students select three guidelines that would be most useful person for them (answers will vary from student to student).

What the peer leader(s) does

- Write the activity on the blackboard (if that method is used).
- Be a group leader and report back to the class (if that method is used).

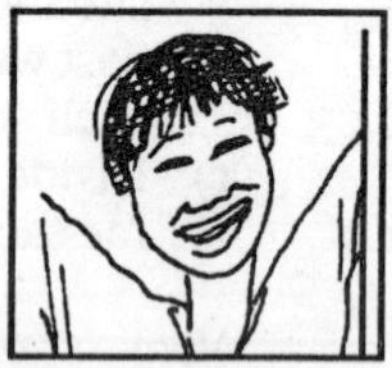

What should be done by parent(s)

(if a Parents' Guide is used):

Students might take this activity home and read and/or discuss the situations and answers with their parents (if each student is given an activity sheet).

Additional preparation

Teachers might want to decide on other (than those given here) acceptable answers for each situation, before doing this activity with students.

2.6. AFFECTION WITHOUT SEX?

Purpose

It is unreasonable to expect young people not to show affection (botl physical and emotional) during this stage of their lives. It is importan to provide alternative activities for those who wish to delay sex.

What the teacher does

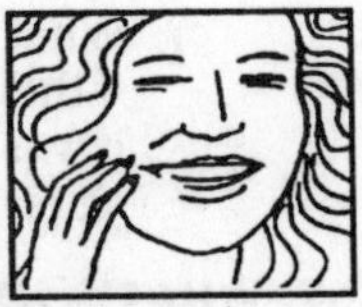

Special concern:

- Students may suggest some physical activities during this exercise that may be diffilcult to talk about, i.e. oral sex, masturbation, petting with or without clothes, body rubbing with or without clothes.
- Be prepared to use local slang with the students.

1. Decide how to teach this strategy.
   a) Form pairs or small groups in the classroom and provide each pair/group with one activity sheet.
   b) Draw the activity on the board and have students work in pairs or small groups to complete the task.

2. Look at ways of showing affection.

Ask the students to look at the list of ways of showing affection shown in the first heart. Then have them discuss in pairs or small groups other ways of showing affection. Their suggestions may be written on the blackboard and the class may discuss together whether or not they are safe and acceptable (i.e. do not put a person at risk for HIV, AIDS/STD). When agreement has been reached on this, the students may write in the second heart their preferred suggestions for ways of showing affection without sex. You might expect some of the more physical affections to include: touch on the shoulder; kissing; open-mouth kissing; petting while clothed (above and below the waist); mutua] masturbation; body-to-body rubbing (clothed and without clothing); oral sex, etc. Students may use quite a different language in trying to express these physical affections.

3. Ask the following questions:
   a) Why is it important for young people to show affection without sex?
      It is important because it: promotes healthy communication; reduces the chance of HIV/STD; reduces the risk of pregnancy; promotes respect for self and partner; reduces the risk of unwanted sex; provides acceptance, warmth and touch to another person and yourself.
   b) Is it important to discuss this topic with a partner? Why or why not? Yes, but it might cause embarrassment or it might end a relationship.

c) What would make it easier to discuss this with a partner? If there was respect, trust and openness in both people; if it was discussed before being in an emotional and sexual situation.

2.7. WHAT'S NEXT?

Purpose

Physical affection can be very sexually arousing. The more sexually arousing the activity is, the more likely it will eventually lead to sex. Establishing limits, and knowing when to express these limits is very important for young people.

> You may want to use the image of the mountain (see students' activities 2.7) in order to illustrate to students that the more physical one gets, the more difficult it is to stop. In this image, sexual arousal is shown as a continuum from least physical to most physical, and students are asked to place various sexual behaviours at different levels on this continuum.

What the teacher does

1. Decide how to teach this activity.
   a) Provide each student with an activity sheet and have them work individually, in pairs or in small groups.
   b) Draw the activity on the blackboard and have a class discussion as to where the various sexual behaviours should be placed (only one activity sheet needed).
   c) Provide one activity sheet for each group and do the activity in small groups.

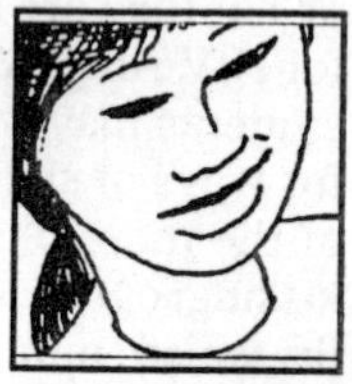

2. Check the answers to the mountain climbing. Explain the concept to the students (see box above).

   1) Holding hands-Least physical
   2) Hugging
   3) Dry kissing
   4) Deep (wet) kissing
   5) Touching breasts and/or genitals on top of clothes
   6) Touching breasts and/or genitals under clothes
   7) Body rubbing with no clothes - Most physical next to sexual intercourse.

3. Discuss the answers to the questions in "Teacher asks".

1) Why is it hard to stop as you get closer physically?
Curiosity and sexual desire put pressure on the couple to move to the next step. It is hard to stop and certainly very difficult to go back a step.
2) Would it be easy to go back to a safer activity?
Why or why not? For most people it would be difficult to go back a step. Strong sexual urges, curiosity and risk-taking would probably lead one to go on rather than back.
3) Where do you think the limit is?
Answers will vary but it is very difficult to stop after 5 or 6. If it has been discussed and agreed upon by both partners not to have sex, then it is possible to set limits.

4) Who should decide where the limit is?
When should this limit be decided? If there is disagreement, one person may have to be very assertive with the other about where they want to stop. The best or safest time to do this is before you become too aroused, but you can stop whenever you feel uncomfortable.

2.8. AM I ASSERTIVE?

Purpose

Being able to describe and recognize verbal and non-verbal aspects of assertive, passive and aggressive behaviour is an important first step in learning how to be assertive oneself.

What the teacher does

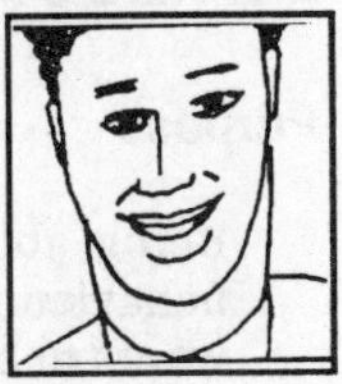

1. Decide how to teach this activity.
   a) Provide the information sheet for each student. Read the words and demonstrate, using body language, the non-verbal aspects of each behaviour.
   b) Put the words "Passive", "Aggressive", "Assertive" on the blackboard and ask students to describe verbal and non-verbal characteristics of each behaviour. Write these under each type of behaviour.

2. You might want to demonstrate or have students demonstrate the verbal and non-verbal aspects of each behaviour- using the verbal and non verbal descriptions on the activity sheet.
3. You could add the following points to your lesson:

Passive behaviour	*Assertive behaviour*	*Aggressive behaviour*
Passive feelings	*Assertive feelings*	*Aggressive feelings*
• helpless	• you feel better about yourself	• angry
• resentful	• self confident	• frustrated
• disappointed	• in control	• bitter
• anxious	• respected by others	• guilty or lonely afterwards
Passive outcomes	Assertive outcomes	Aggressive outcomes
• you don't get what you want	• you don't hurt others	• you dominate
• anger builds up	• you gain respect for yourself	• you humiliate
• you feel lonely	• your rights and others' are respected	• you win at the expense of others
• rights are violated	• you both win	

What the peer leader(s) does

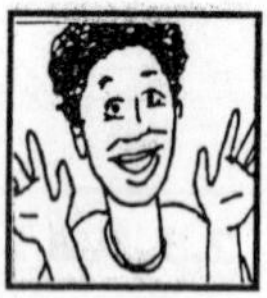

Peer leaders could be very helpful in suggesting additional characteristie these three types of behaviour; and in demonstrating the three type behaviours.

Additional preparation

Set up a role-play with your peer leaders that would demonstrate these three types of behaviours.

2.9. WHO'S ASSERTIVE?

Purpose

Being able to recognize assertive, passive and aggressive behaviour in real-life situations is important for a person who wants to be assertive.

What the teacher does

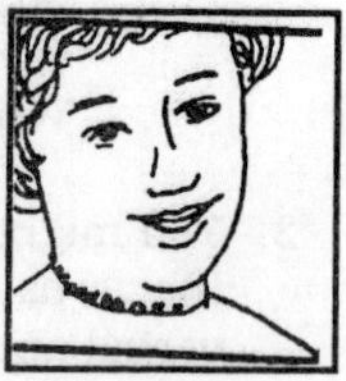

1. Decide how to teach this activity.
   a) Provide an activity sheet for each student and have the students work on the activity individually, in pairs or in small groups.
   b) Read the two stories and ask the students to identify the behaviours of

the three people in the stories (only one activity sheet is needed).

c) Place the students in groups and give out one activity sheet for each group.

2. Give the students the answers to the questions about the three people in the stories.

• ***Story 1***

Rob's behaviour is:	Passive
Why?	
What said?	"I knov. you'll think I'm crazy........." "Well, OK, I'll go".
How said?	Soft voice; low voice.
Body position?	Head down; hangs his head; eyes down; defeated.
Sulana's behaviour is:	Aggressive
Why?	
What said?	"You are crazy and not only that but you're stupid too".
How said?	Interrupts; loudly.
Body position?	Nose to nose; hands on hips.

• ***Story 2***

Tana's behaviour is:	Assertive
Why?	
What said?	"Could we talk where no one is around" (privacy); Asks for feedback and takes other person's feelings into account.
How said?	Calm but firm.
Body position?	Sits straight; looks person in the eye.

3. If time permits, ask students to role-play these two scenes.

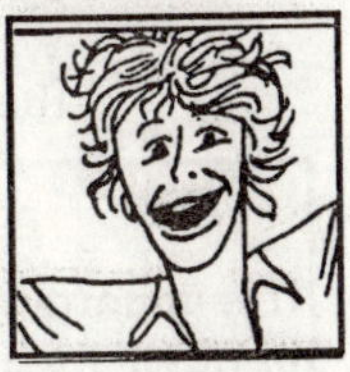

What the peer leader(s) does

The peer leaders could:

- Work with a small group
- Role-play the two stories
- Write on the blackboard

Additional preparation

Teachers might want to prepare peer leaders to do a role-play of the two situations.

2.10. ASSERTIVE MESSAGES

Purpose

It is important for students to learn the specific steps in being assertive and to practise these steps through behavioural rehearsal.

What the teacher does

1. Decide how to teach this activitv.
   a) Provide an activity sheet for each student so that they can follow the four steps to an assertive message.
   b) Write the four steps with the "words you might say" on the blackboard. Thens with another student (peer leader) role-play the situation described (only two activity sheets are needed).

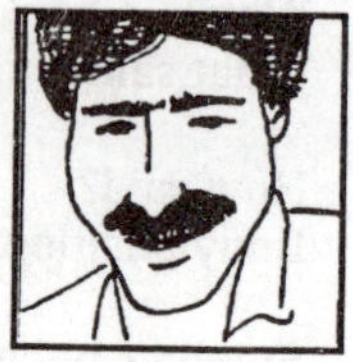

2. Explain the four steps and the words that might be used, to the students. Point out that steps 3 and 4 - asking how the other person feels anu thanking the other person - are ways of respecting and being assertivt with that person.
3. Read the situation for the role-play and then act out the assertive message with another student (peer leader). Emphasize that in this role-play the person who is replying is accepting the assertive person's message.

What the peer leader(s) does

Peer leaders should be able to:

- Help the teacher in the role-play by being the person who replies to the assertive message.
- Write the activity on the blackboard (if this method is used).

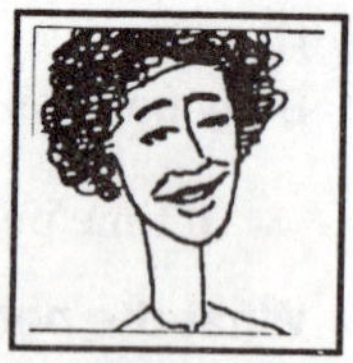

Additional preparation

It is important to practise this assertive message with peer leaders or other students before you demonstrate to the students.

2.11. YOUR ASSERETIVE MESSAGE

Purpose

By preparing an assertive message with the whole class, it is easier students to prepare their own assertive message during the next activity.

What the teacher does

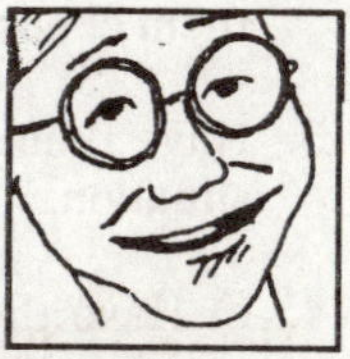

1. Decide how you are going to do this activity:
   a) Provide each student with an activity sheet and have them fill in the "bubbles you do the activity with the whole class.
   b) Put the activity on the blackboard and fill in the "bubbles" with the suggestions from the class (only one activity sheet needed).
   c) Place students in small groups and provide each group with an activity sheet have the group develop ideas for step 1 and then ask for suggestions from each group. Select the best suggestion and have the recorder from each group enter step in the "bubble". Do the same for steps 2, 3, 4.
2. Read the situation at the top of the page. Also read step 1.
3. Ask students for suggestions for the first "bubbl..". Take the best one and have the students write this on their activity sheet.
4. Do the same for steps 2, 3, response of the other person and step 4.
5. When the message is finished, role-play the message with a student play the part of Adula.

What the peer leader(s) does

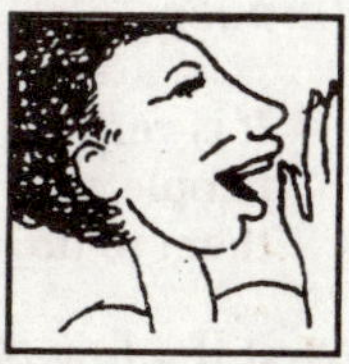

Peer leaders could:

- Be in charge of a small group
- Role-play the developed message with the teacher or another peer leader

2.12. YOUR ASSERTIVE MESSAGE

Purpose

Students are given the opportunity to develop and practise their own assertive message.

What the teacher does

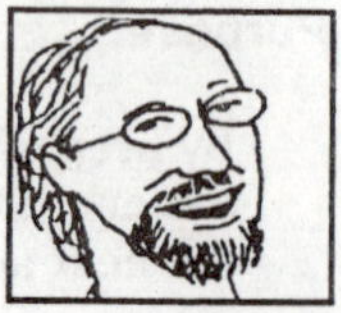

1. Decide how to teach this activity:
   a) Provide an activity sheet for each student in the class and have them write ou assertive message individually or preferably in pairs.
   b) Divide the students into small groups and provide one activity sheet per groups.

2. Either assign a situation (there are four) to the students or let them choose their own.

3. Have them write out an assertive message for their chosen situation.

4. a) Have the groups role-play the situations they have been assignes have chosen.

   b) Ask for volunteers to role-play their script in front of the class. Look for verbal and non-verbal aspects of their message. Be very positiv they volunteer.

What the peer leader(s) does

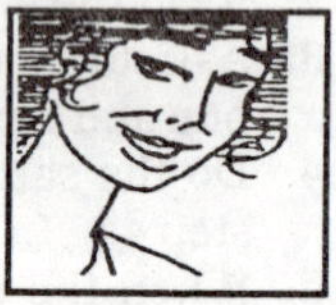

Peer leaders could:
- Volunteer to role-play their script
- Lead a small group (if working in groups)

2.13. RESPONDING TO PERSUASION

Purpose

It is very important that students learn to deal assertively with people who try to distract or pressure them by persuading them to do some thing they do not think they should.

What the teacher does

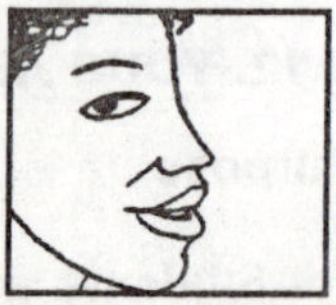

1. Decide how to teach this activity.
   a) Provide a copy to each student to follow as you go over each section.
   b) Read the various parts of the activity, putting the important parts on the black board, i.e., the ways to "get back on topic" and to "refuse", "delay", or "bargain

2. Read "Ways people get you off the message or do not accept it". Role-play each line, e.g. "You're just afraid." Ask the students to provide other lines similar to the one read.
3. Show the students how to "Get back on topic" if they are distracted. for additional ways.
4. Show the students ways to "refuse", "delay", and "bargain".

What the peer leader(s) does

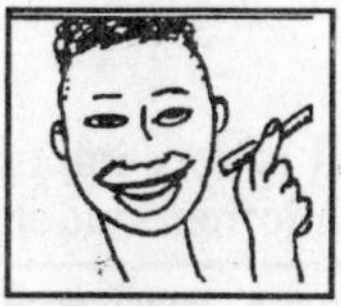

The peer leaders should be able to:

- Role-play the parts or lines used by the teacher in his/her explanation
- Put the activity on the blackboard.

Additional preparation

Teachers should read this activity carefully and decide how they might demonstrate the various sections.

RESPONDING TO PERSUASION

Purpose

Students need to know the techniques of an assertive message when someone is trying to distract them or persuade them to do something they don't want to do.

What the teacher does

1. Decide how to teach this activity.
   a) Provide an activity sheet for each student in the class. Let them follow you as explain the activity.
   b) Read the activity and put important parts on the blackboard, e.g. the lines to order to refuse, delay and bargain.

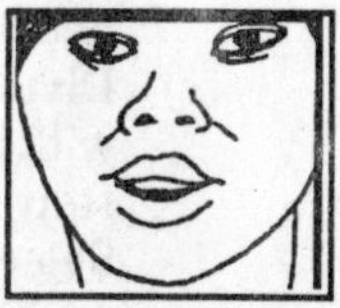

2. Read each step and the persuader's statements and responses. After each step, statement or response, role-play the words in the "bubble". example, step 1 - Explain your feelings and the problem: "I feel scared about driving with you when you have been drinking."
3. When you have finished each step, role-play the entire assertive sage once more, using a student volunteer (peer leader) to play the of the older brother. Do the role-play three times, using a different ending (refuse, delay, bargain) each time.

What the peer leader(s) does

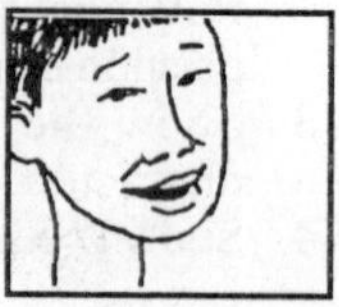

Peer leaders should be able to help you by:

- Role-playing the situation with you
- Writing information on the blackboard
- Explaining the refuse, delay, and bargain endings

Additional preparation

It is very important to practise this script with a peer leader(s) or another student before demonstrating it in front of your class.

2.14. RESPONDING TO PERSUASION

Purpose

An example of distraction and persuasion makes it easier for students to learn to deal with these problems and develop their own strategies.

What the teacher does

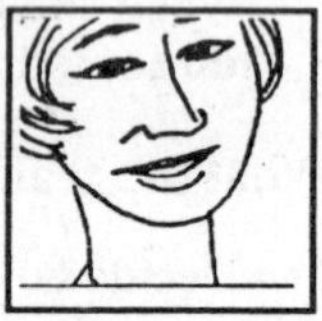

1. Decide how to teach this activity
   a) Provide each student with an activity sheet and have them fill in the "bubbles" as you the activity with the whole class.
   b) Put the activity on the blackboard and fill in the "bubbles" with the suggestions from class (only one activity sheet needed).
   c) Divide students into small groups and provide each group with an activity sheet. Have the group develop ideas for step I and then ask for suggestions from each group. Select the best suggestion and have the recorder from each group enter that step in the "bub provided. Do the same for the other steps and responses in the activity.
2. Read the situation at the top of the page. Also read step one and words that might be used.
3. Ask students for suggestions for step 1 and select the best one. Hav students put this in the first "bubble" on their activity sheet.
4. Do the same for the remaining steps and responses.
5. When the message is finished, role-play it with a volunteer student (or peer leader) three times using a different ending (refuse, delay, or bargain) each time.
6. Discuss the question; different answers are possible.

What the peer leader(s) does

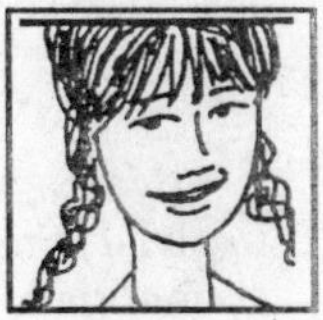

The peer leaders should be able to:
- Role-play with the teacher
- Be in charge of a small group
- Write the activity on the blackborad

2.15. RESPONDING TO PERSUASION

Purpose

Students learn how to deal with distracting statements and how to be assertive when someone is pressuring them to do something they do not want to do.

What the teacher does

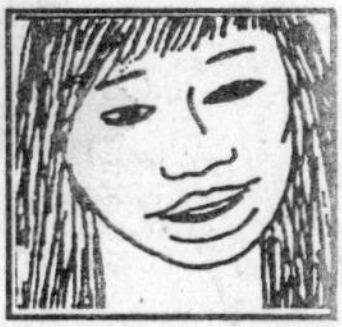

1. Decide how to teach this activity.

   a) Provide an activity sheet for each student in the class and have them write out an assertive message to a distracting and persuading person, individually or preferably in pairs.

   b) Place the students in small groups and provide one activity sheet for each group.

2. Either assign a situation (there are three) to the students or let them choose their own.

3. Have them write out an assertive message for the situation they have chosen, in the "bubbles" (as in the class activity).

4. They should read it to themselves, make changes and then read it once more.

5. Tell the students that they may be asked to role-play their situation in front of the class.

What the peer leader(s) does

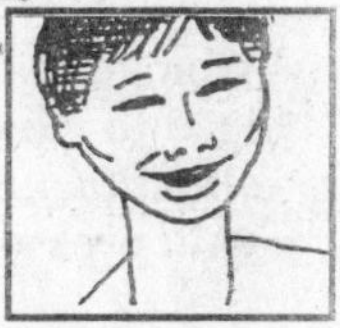

The peer leaders can help you by:
- Volunteering to role-play his or her script
- Leading a small group (if working in groups)

2.16. YOU DECIDE

Purpose

Boys/men often have different ideas about delaying sex from girls/ women. Most of these are old ideas and need to be changed.

What the teacher does

1. Decide how to teach this activity.
   a) Provide an activity for each student and have them do the activity individually, in pairs or in small groups.
   b) Read the statement. Ask the students to indicate if they agree or disagree. (Only one activity sheet is needed.)
   c) Put the students in small groups and have them complete the activity (one sheet per group needed).

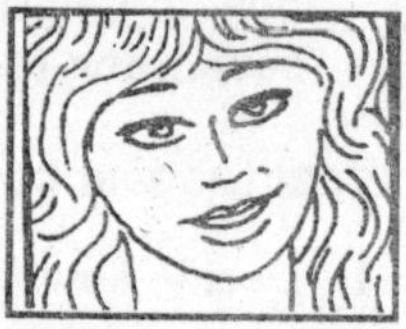

2. You will have to explain to the students that they should indicate "agree" if, generally speaking, they think the statement is correct or right for themselves, and "disagree" if they think that this is not the right way of thinking or this idea is incorrect or wrong.
3. Next, the students are asked to change the old statements into new ones by completing the unfinished statements.
4. After the students have completed the activity you should conduct a class discussion. The agree-disagree can be clarified by a show of hands. Ask students to volunteer their answers to the unfinished sentences.
5. Ask students to suggest new statements and choose the one that receives wide consensus.

2.17. DEALING WITH THREATS AND VIOLENCE

Purpose

Women, particularly, need to be aware of situations that may lead to violent sex and of people who may put them in those situations. They also need to learn ways of avoiding or dealing with pressures and threats to have sex.

What the teacher does

1. Decide how to teach this activity:

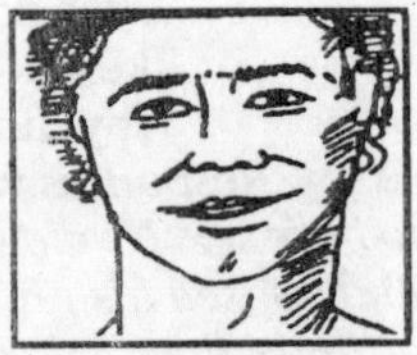

a) Provide each student with an activity sheet and have them work individually, in pairs or in small groups.
b) Read the story to the students and ask the questions under "Teacher asks."
c) Form small groups and provide each group with one activity sheet to use for discussion.

2. Discuss the questions with the students. Possible answers are suggested below.
   1) Do you think that Maria could have been aware of what was going to happen? What were the clues that could have told her?
   Yes. Walking alone on a possibly deserted country road; Carlos flirting and talking about sex; going into an abandoned house; touching her.
   2) Maria was silent and embarrassed when Carlos started talking about sex. What could she have done instead of being silent and embarrassed?
   She probably should have been assertive and told him that she did not like what he was doing and that she was going home.
   3) What should she do now? Keep it a secret? Tell someone she trusts (parents, teachers, religious leader)? Should she talk to Carlos about the matter? What might happen if she doesn't tell anyone about the situation?
   She has to make her own decision but generally it is a good idea to talk to someone she trusts. Whether she should tell the police and/or go to a hospital should be discussed with that person. She should arrange to be tested for STD/HIV (and pregnancy if necessary). It is not likely that anything can be accomplished by talking to Carlos. She may feel unnecessarily ashamed, lonely and worried if she doesn't tell anyone.
   4) List things you can do to help prevent violence and threats:
      a. When you're with someone who suggests having sex and you don't want to.
      Be assertive and tell the person in a firm manner that you are not interested. Leave with a friend.
      If possible, move to where there are other people. Phone someone if phones are available.
      b. When someone becomes physical and tries to force you to have sex.
      Scream; fight; kick in the testicles only if you can get away quickly; delay; bargain depending on the situation (if your life is threatened or a weapon is being used). Be very assertive.

5) What do you think about Carlos? Are there other men like Carlos? What should he have done in this situation? Why did he do what he did?

Responses will vary. If at all in doubt, he should not have tried to have sex. He did what he did because: he lacked respect for women and abused his physical power over Maria; he had a common male attitude that "no" doesn't really mean "no"; and perhaps because she agreed to go for a walk alone. with him in the country.

2.18. BEING ASSERTIVE EVERY DAY

Purpose

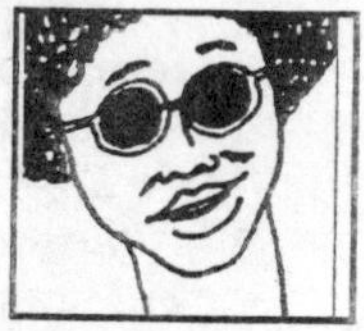

There is a need to transfer the skills that are taught in the classroom to everyday life. Therefore, it is important for the student to learn to be assertive in his/her daily activities.

What the teacher does

1. The teacher explains to the students how this activity is done. Have the students develop their plan at school and practise it at home. Here are a few key points that you should emphasize:
   - Tell the students the purpose of the activity - there is no sense in learning how to be assertive in the classroom if you don't apply what you have learned to your everyday life.
   - Explain that the "Personal plan" is a way of carrying out your plan, a contract with yourself and finally an evaluation of how you did.
   - Have them select an assertive goal - get them to make their goal specific, for example, "to say how I feel when Susan puts me down." Goals can include: handling criticism; giving compliments; asking a favour; showing you are hurt; giving your own opinion; making new friends; saying "no" to something, etc.
   - The dates should also be specific, for example, "start on Monday, July 1 at 9 a.m. and finish on Sunday, July 7 at 6 p.m."
   - Benefits should also be specific rather than general. "I will probably feel better about myself (self-respect); get what I need, and still not hurt my friend."
   - Rewards can include many things - food, drinks, a trip, buying something, a holiday, telling someone special about what you did, etc.

- If the student signs a contract with her/himself, she/he is more likely to complete the task. Sometimes having a friend sign as a witness further reinforces the student's motivation.
- Identifying obstacles that may get in the way of reaching a person's goal can be of help, if plans are made in advance, in overcoming these problems.

What should be done by parent(s)

(if a Parents' Guide is used)

It would be useful for students to inform their parents of their action plan so that parents could help students follow through with their assertive message. Students could take their personal plan home and discuss it with their parents.

Additional preparation

Students should be advised to try their assertive message with someone who is likely to be positive about their being assertive (i.e. avoid someone who might get angry or violent).

Unit 3

Responsible Behaviour: Protected Sex

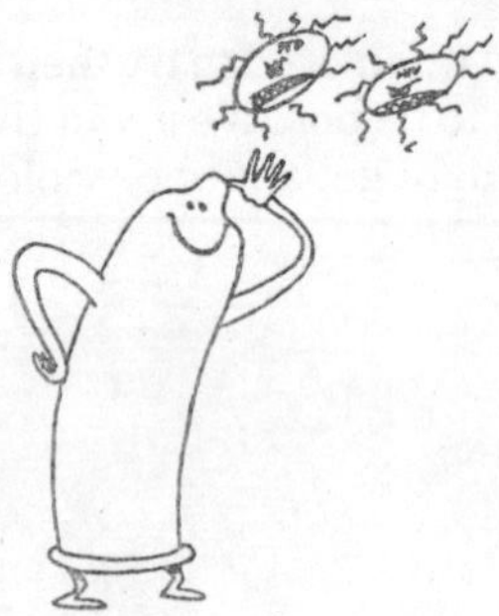

3.1. THE CONDOM

Purpose

Information about condoms is necessary for effective use.

What the teacher does

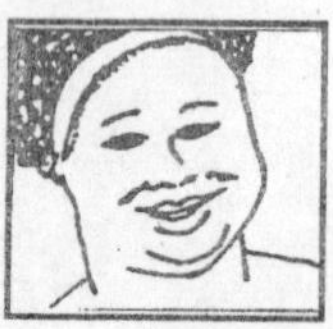

1. Provide an activity sheet for each student or read the questions and answer to the students.
2. Emphasis should be placed on the fact that condoms are strong, safe sensitive and easy to use.
   Remind students that Vaseline and other oil-based lubricants should not be used they weaken latex condoms. Only water-based lubricants such as K-jelly, glycerine egg white, spermicidal jelly or foam, MuKo and Lubafax should be used.

3. Ask if there are any questions about condoms and provide answers you can. If not, tell the students you will find the answer for the next day.

3.2. ARGUMENTS PEOPLE USE AGAINST USING CONDOMS

Purpose

A person may be very positive about condom use but may have a partner who does not like condoms and doesn't want to use them. It is important to learn how to talk to a person who dis'ịkes using condoms.

What the teacher does

1. Decide how you will use this activity.
   a) Provide an activity sheet for each student in the class and have them work individually or in pairs to complete the instructions.
   b) Read the "Arguments against" and give the three responses to the argument. Students choose what they think is the best response and write down the letter of the response (only one activity sheet is needed).
   c) Place the students in small groups and have the students make a group decision on the best response (one sheet per group is needed).

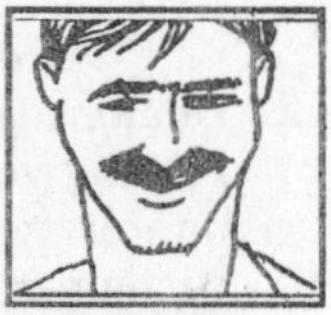

2. Ask for responses to each argument. It is best if you can have one student make the argument and another read their chosen response. For example, one student would say, "They spoil the mood", and the other responds, "Hey, condoms may even be fun".

3.3/4. HOW TO USE A CONDOM (CONDOM PRACTICE)

Purpose

One of the most important factors in condom failure is inexperience with its proper use. Therefore, a demonstration of its actual use is imnortant.

What the teacher does

- The teacher should explain to students that at first they might feel awkward but that these feelings pass with practice. If something humorous occurs, enjoy the moment (but don't accept put-downs).

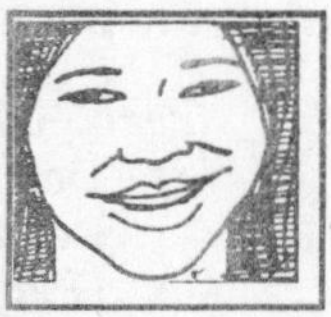

- The teacher should inform the class that this is an optional activity.
  However, he/she should indicate to students that the reason for doing this activity is to acquire a skill that may be needed in the future. It is not taught to encourage sex and it is not an invitation to seek sex.
- It may be difficult for students to volunteer for this activity. To avoid embarrassment, it is suggested that the teacher select one or two students (or the peer leaders) to practise. The rest of the class can practise afterwards.
- Give support and positive feedback to the students practicing using a condom.

1. Decide how to teach this activity.
   a) Provide each student with an activity sheet to follow the steps of effective condom use.
   b) Divide students into small groups and assign a peer leader to each group (one activity sheet needed per group).
2. Demonstrate how to use a condom with a student (peer leader) helping you by reading each step as you do it. (You will need one or two condoms and a model penis or a banana or a cucumber; alternatively students can practise on their fingers.) If time permits, change positions with the student and read the steps while the student (peer leader) demonstrates.
3. If the class is divided into small groups, ask the peer leaders to demonstrate condom use to their group and encourage all students to practise themselves.
   The peer leaders may have to have had prior instruction.
4. Discuss questions with students (under Teacher asks). Students may share what they have heard about experience with condoms.

Note:

1. *Humour is important. A relaxed class atmosphere is important.*
2. *It is alright to make mistakes. It shows that students too can make mistakes while practising.*
3. *Having a student demonstrate is the best learning situation as peers will listen and follow their classmates more than they do their teachers.*
4. *You may need someone to hold the banana, cucumber or model penis (you need two hands).*

What the peer leader(s) does

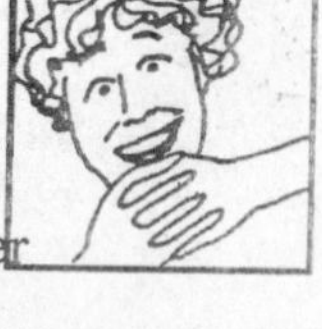

Peer leaders could help you:

- Demonstrate
- Read the steps in effective condom use
- Hold the model penis, banana or cucumber

3.5. NO TO UNPROTECTED SEX

Purpose

Using the skills learned in Unit 2 on assertive behaviour, students lets to use an assertive message with a partner who doesn't want to us condom or doesn't have one to use.

What the teacher does

1. Decide how to teach this activity:
   a) Provide each student with an activity sheet and have them follow the script as teacher reviews the steps and role-plays the situation.
   b) Review the steps and role-play the situation with another student (only two active sheets are needed).

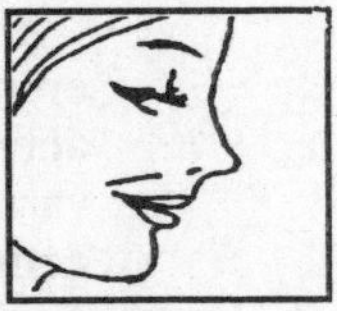

2. Have a student (peer leader) read each step as you (or another stude read the script.
3. Do the role-play three times - first with a refuse ending, then a depending, and finally with a bargain ending. You may want to use different students for the second and third role-play.
4. Tell them that the next step is for the whole class to develop the the different endings.

What the peer leader(s) does

Peer leaders can help the teacher by:
- Playing a role in the situation with the teacher.
- Role-playing an ending with another student (peer leader).

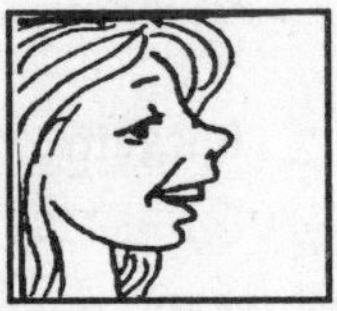

3.6. NO TO UNPROTECTED SEX

Purpose

To provide the class with an opportunity to make an assertive response to a person who has negative attitudes towards condoms and is persuading a person to have sex without a condom.

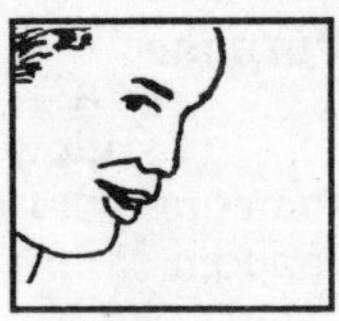

What the teacher does

1. Decide how to teach this activity:

a) Provide each student with an activity sheet. The teacher will read or role-play the situatio and students will suggest refuse, delay, and bargain responses. The students and teacher wii decide on the best response and put it in the appropriate space.

b) The teacher will do the activity in a similar way as a) but the students will not have an activity sheet. Responses will be written on the blackboard and students will write the best response on a piece of paper (only one activity sheet is needed).

c) Students are placed in small groups and one activity sheet is provided for each group. The group makes suggestions on responses and the best response is recorded. A class activity follows in which the best response from the various groups is recorded on the blackboard (only one activity sheet per group is needed).

2. Suggestions for refuse, delay and bargain responses are obtained from the students and the best response is recorded.
3. When completed, role-play the total scene three times - using refusal for the first time, delay the second and bargain the third time. The teacher and, student (peer leader) or two students (two peer leaders) can do the role play. An example is shown below of a possible refuse, delay and bargan ending.

Refuse: You know I like you very much but I really don't want to have sex without a condom.

Delay: I think it would be a good idea to wait until you feel less embarrassed about condom

Bargain: Maybe we could buy condoms together and I could help you use one.

What the peer leader(s) does

Peer leaders can:

- Be in charge of a small group.
- Role-play the situation.

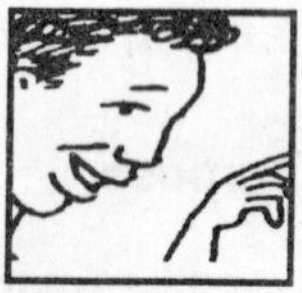

3.7. NO TO UNPROTECTED SEX

Purpose

To allow students to make their own assertive responses to someone who is trying to persuade them to have sex without a condom.

What the teacher does

1. Decide how to teach this activity.

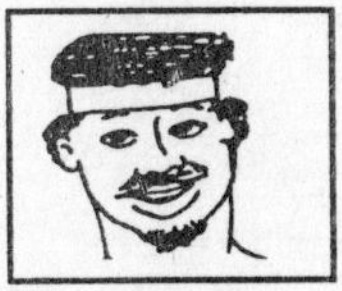

a) Provide an activity sheet for each student and have them do the activity individually or in pairs.
b) Read the situation and response and have the students write their refuse, delay and bargain ending on a piece of paper (only one activity sheet needed).
c) Write the activity on the blackboard and have the students write their refuse, delay and bargain ending on a piece of paper (one activity sheet needed).

2. Ask the students to read out their suggestions for the three endings.
3. Ask for volunteers to read the entire script with a different ending each time. Examples of the three endings are provided below.

Refuse:	Even though I'd like to have sex with you, I definitely won't without a condom.
Delay:	It can't hurt to wait until we do have a condom. I'll feel so much safer.
Bargain:	Let's just fool around this time and have sex when we do have a condom.

What the peer leader(s) does

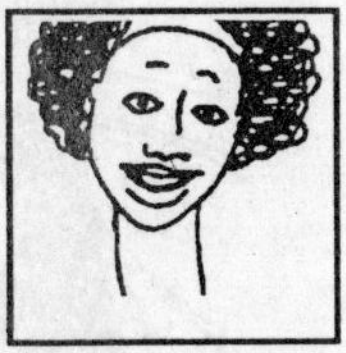

Peer leaders can:

- Write the activity on the blackboard.
- Role-play the three endings.

Unit 4

Care and Support

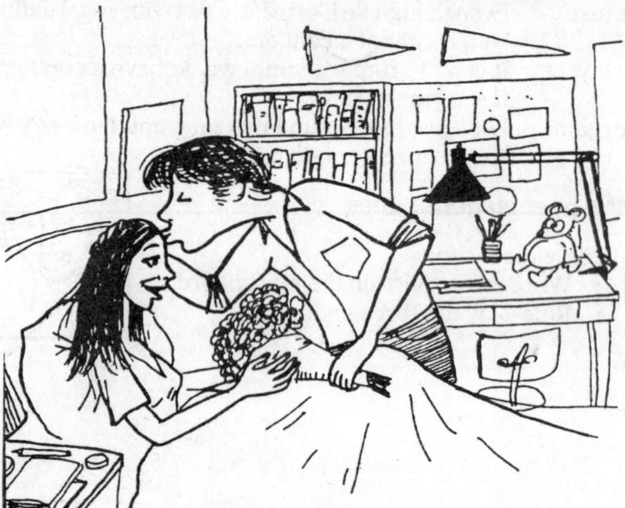

4.1. WHO DISCRIMINATES?

Purpose

People who are HIV-positive or who are living with AIDS are often subject to discrimination. Young people need to be aware of discrimination and how it is expressed.

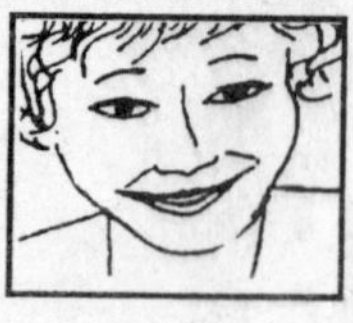

What the teacher does

1. Decide how to teach this activity:

a) Provide each student with an activity sheet and have them work individually or in pairs to complete the activity.

b) Read the definition and examples of discrimination. Then read the four quotes and have the students complete the unfinished sentences verbally, on a sheet of paper or on the blackboard (only one activity sheet is needed).

c) Place the students in small groups and provide one activity sheet per group. Have the group complete the instructions.

2. Have the students complete the unfinished sentences. Suggested answers are given below:

• ***School discrimination***

A person who has HIV infection is not allowed to attend school.

This is wrong because: A person with HIV or AIDS can pass the virus to someone else only through sexual intercourse, transfer of blood products, or from mother tc baby. There is no danger of transmission by day-to-day social contact.

• ***The village banning***

The Council will not allow people with AIDS to live in the village.

This is wrong because: It discriminates against a person's rights with no reason aq the virus cannot be transmitted through daily activities, or by living near to a persor with AIDS.

• ***Work in the fruit stand***

Mancini, the owner of the fruit stand won't allow Harsi, who has HIV infection, to work for him.

This is wrong because: Again, this is discrimination. The owner obviously does no know how HIV is transmitted and perhaps he is afraid he won't get business if other people. know that Harsi has HIV infection.

• ***A government decision***

The government has decided not to allow people with HIV to enter the country. This will not stop AIDS because: there are many, many people with HIV who do not know they have the virus and are already in the country. Therefore it discriminates against those who have been tested.

Remember: testing everybody is not an effective method to stop the infection, and can lead to a sense of false security because:

- The test would need to be repeated very often for all the population
- People would find a way to get false certificates
- One can get infected immediately after obtaining a HIV-negative test result

3. Discuss the questions under "Teacher asks". Suggested answers are found below.
   a) Why do people discriminate?
      - They learn from parents, adults and their peers
      - Lack of accurate information
      - Fear of certain kinds of people
      - Dislike of anyone who is different b) Why is it important not to discriminate?
      - It hurts other people
      - It isn't fair
      - We wouldn't want to be treated that way
      - Equality is a fundamental human right

   c) What could you do if you heard discriminating remarks about a person witE HIV infection or AIDS from someone in your community?
      - Inform the person that they are wrong and tell them why. Be assertive and tell th person you do not want to hear their comments.
      - Explain why it is important to be compassionate and supportive to someone wit} HIV infection or AIDS.

Invite a person with HIV infection or AIDS, or a relative, to talk to the classroom; it will be a profound experience for you and the students.

4.2. THE STORY OF TWO COMMUNITIES

Purpose

It is important for young people to feel what it is like to be discriminated against. This can be at least partially accomplished by reflecting on comments made by a person living with AIDS. This is a true story only the names have been changed.

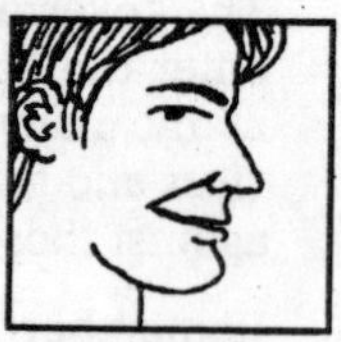

What the teacher does

1. Decide how to teach this activity:
   a) Provide each student with an activity sheet and have the students work individually or in pairs to complete the activity.

b) Read the comments and actions from community A and community B once. Read them a second time and have the students individually decide on the three most hurtful and three most helpful and to explain why they chose those three. Ask the students to write a couple of sentences about how they feel about community A and about community B. (Only one activity sheet needed.)

2. Ask students to identify the three most hurtful and the three most helpful comments and to explain their choices. Then ask them about their feelings about community A and community B.
3. Finally, discuss the question at the end of the activity. Answers are suggested below:

Why do you think there was such a difference between the two communities?

- Ignorance about transmission in cornmunity A
- Fear on the part of a large group of people
- Education programme in comrnunity B
- Peers supporting Ryando

What should be done by parent(s)
(if a Parents' Guide is used)

This would be an excellent activity for students to take home to their parents. Students could compare their 3 answers for each community with those that their parents selected. (Students could read the comments if parents are unable to read.)

4.3. WHY COMPASSION?

People who have compassion towards themselves and others are very groups much needed in this society. Understanding why compassion is important is the first step.

What the teacher does

1. Decide how to teach this activity.
   a) Provide an activity sheet for each student and have them complete the activity individually, in pairs, or in small groups.

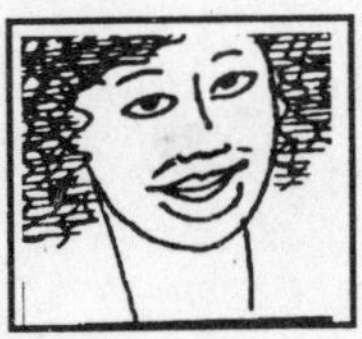

   b) Read the three reasons for being compassionate and ask students for other reasons. Add these to the list. Then ask students to select the two that are most important to them (only one activity sheet is needed).

c) Place the students in small groups and provide one activity sheet for each group. Have them add to the list and then each group member selects the two that are most important to them.

2. Ask the students for other reasons for being compassionate. Add these to the list. Some possibilities might be:
   - We have a moral duty to care for sick people
   - They are a minority and are therefore discriminated against
   - They are often rejected by people who care for the sick
   - They are often very young to be dying
   - They are often rejected by family and friends
   - It feels nice to help or care for someone
   - It will help you overcome your own fears of death and AIDS
3. Discuss the question under "Teacher asks". Suggested answers are provided below:

Why is it difficult for some people to show compassion?

- They have had a lot of pain themselves and are only able to look after themselves
- They only think about themselves
- They don't know how to be compassionate
- They are afraid to be compassionate

4.4. WHAT COULD YOU DO?

Purpose It is important to know of ways to be compassionate and when and how to help.

What the teacher does

1. Decide on a method to teach this activity:

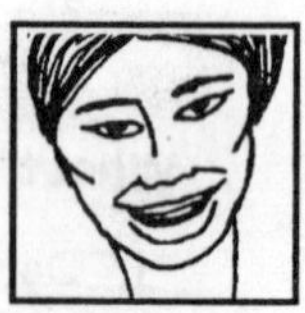

   a) Provide each student with an activity sheet and have them complete the activity individually or in pairs.

   b) Write the stories on the blackboard and have the students complete the activity individually or in pairs (only one activity sheet needed).

   c) Place the students in small groups and give each group one activity sheet. The groups must reach a consensus on the ways to help Minori and Dwari.
2. Allow the students to suggest other ways of being compassionate. Have them place these in the blank spaces on the "Helping heart".
3. Ask for suggestions for ways to help with Minori's heart and Dwari's heart. Ask students to explain their choice.

4. Answer the question under "Teacher asks". Suggested answers are provided below:

What would be most difficult for you if a friend or relative of yours had AIDS?

Responses will vary but they may include: the death of a loved one; the pain and depression many will experience; the loss of health and vitality; the changes in appearance; the loss of control of bodily functions

What would be most difficult for the person with AIDS?

Responses may include: acting naturally; sharing emotions (laughing, crying); celebrating special days without showing despair.

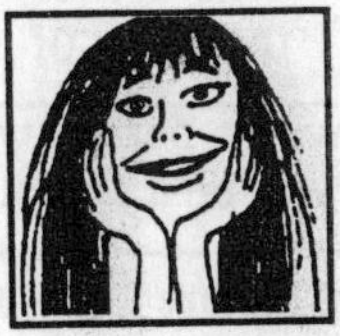

What the peer leader(s) does

Peer leaders could help by:

- Putting the activity on the blackboard
- Being in charge of a small group
- Volunteering answers to various questions

What should be done by parent(s)

(if a Parents' Guide is used)

This would be an excellent activity for students to take home and complete with parents. Students could pick their 4 "helps" and parents could do same and they could explain to each other why they chose the ones they did.

4.5. HOW TO'S OF CAREGIVING?

Purpose

Students may be living with a family member who has AIDS, or may know an HIV-infected person in their neighbourhood. It is important that they know how to give emotional and medical help to this person.

What the teacher does

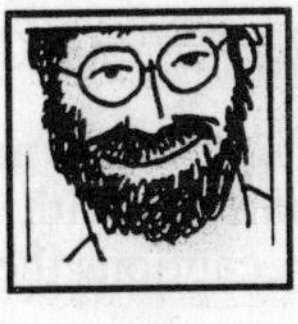

1. Decide how to teach this activity:
   a) Provide each student with an activity sheet and discuss the points made on the sheet. It might be important to have the

students bring this sheet home to their parents (for parents who are helping someone with AIDS).

b) Read the points to the students (only one activity sheet needed).

2. You might ask if anyone in the class is caring for a person with AIDS. If so, they may be able to contribute valuable information and experiences.
3. You may invite a person with AIDS to talk to the class.

What should be done by parent(s)

(if a Parents' Guide is used)

This activity is in the parents' guide and students could read the ways of providing caregiving to their parents.

Invite a person with HIV or AIDS, or a relative, to talk to the class; it will be a profound expenence for you and the students.

4.6. HOW TO KEEP YOUSELF SAFE?

Purpose

It is important for individuals who are caring for people with AIDS to know basic hygiene and home care to protect themselves from HIV.

What the teacher does

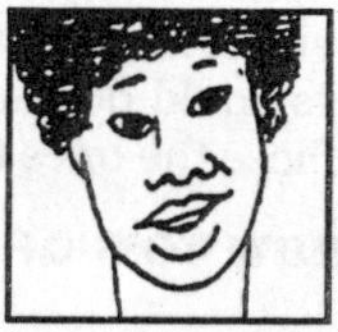

1. Decide how to teach this activity.
   a) Provide an activity sheet for each student and have them follow the points as you read them. This would be a good activity sheet to send home with students for parents who might be caring for someone who has AIDS.
   b) Read the points to the students (only one activity sheet needed).
2. Ask students to read the points under each heading.

What should be done by parent(s)

(if a Parents' Guide is used)

This is an important activity for parents who are looking after someone with HIV or AIDS. They should be aware of the health precautions they need to take to remain healthy.

4.7. WHAT DO YOU KNOW?

Purpose

To review and check information on caregiving (Unit 4 - Activity 5).

What the teacher does

1. Decide how to teach this activity:
   a) Provide an activity sheet for each student and have them complete the acti vity following the instructions.
   b) Put test 1 on the blackboard and read test 2 The students decide on the correct answer for each test (only one activity sheet is needed)
   c) Place students in small groups and provide one activity sheet for each grroup. They decide as a group which are the correct answers

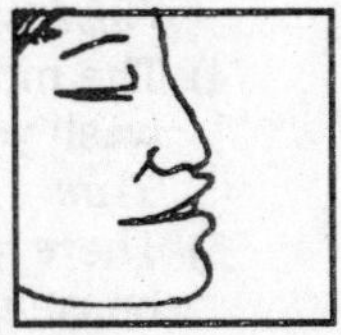

Note: Tests 1 and 2 may be done as a team competition. The class can be divided into two teams with captains and half the questions can be given to team 1 and half to team 2. If small groups are used, they can do both tests an the group with the highest score is the winner.

2. Give the students the correct answers. These are provided below:

Test about caregiving - matching

- A good caregiver is one who is a...
  d) friend and companion
- A person with AIDS who has "sweats", vomiting or diarrhoea needs...
  c) extra fluids
- To stop nausea and vomiting it is best to give...
  f) small meals with little fat
- For a person who is in bed a lot you should...
  h) change their sleeping position
- As a good caregiver you should also...
  b) look after yourself
- You may encourage people who are sad and depressed to express their feelings if they...
  a) become angry or cry
- People who are ill need to do...
  g) what they can for themselves
- The most important skill in being a good caregiver is to...
  e) really listen

True - false statements

1) Latex or rubber gloves should be used when touching body fluids.
   True
2) Injection needles should be put in a plastic bag.
   False: in a plastic or metal box
3) Thermometers can be used more than once without washing.
   False: wash with soap and water every time
4) The most important thing in looking after yourself is to wash your hands with soap and warm water.
   True
5) There have been no HIV infections from living in the same house as a person who has HIV infection or AIDS.
   True
6) Soiled things should be put in a paper bag and then put in the garbage.
   False: double plastic bag
7) It is very important to cover sores, cuts and rashes.
   True
8) You should wash the bathroom with bleach solution that is 1 part bleach to 20 parts water.
   False: 1 part bleach to 10 parts water

3. Have students total their scores for Test 1 and Test 2 and look up their rating score (at the end of the activity).

What should be done by parent(s)

(if a Parents' Guide is used)

This activity is part of the Parents' Guide and after doing Unit 4 - Activity 4 students and parents could do the test to see how much they remember. (If reading ability is a problem, students could read the questions and possible answers to their parents.)

4.8. SUPPORT FOR RESPONSIBLE BEHAVIOUR

Purpose

It is important to encourage young people to support peers who: value abstinence, have made the decision to use a condom, or show tolerance and compassion to people with AIDS.

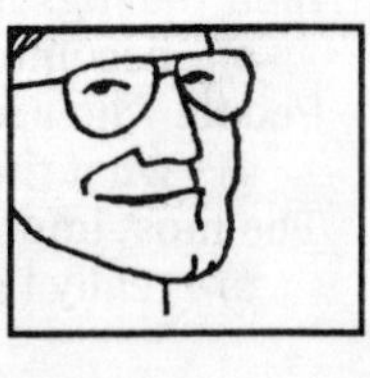

What the teacher does

1. Decide how to teach this activity:

a) Provide an activity sheet for each student and have them work individually or in pairs to complete the activity.
b) Read the four situations to the students and have them decide on support statements that they can make (only one activity sheet is needed).
c) Divide the students into small groups and give one activity sheet to each group. Have the group decide on one or more support statements for each situation.

2. Ask students to read their support statements. Suggestions for each story are provided below:

• ***Story A - A decision not to have sex***

"I really think you made a good decision. If he really loved you he wouldn't pressure you like that."

• ***Story B - No sex without a condom***

"That must have been a tough decision but I think you made the right one - with AIDS and STD you can never be sure."

• ***Story C - To go to the candy store or not***

"Look, people live with, eat, touch and hug people with AIDS and there hasn't been one reported case of transmission this way. We have nothing to worry about. I' d like to go."

• ***Story D - Who do you support***

"You're taking a chance with AIDS around. I hope you know what you're doing."

3. Take up the questions in "Teacher asks". Suggested answers are provide below:
   1) Why do many young people feel it is not "cool" to support healthy decision?
      - It is "cool" to take risks - even those that involve health and safety
      - Some people need to be "macho" to draw attention to themselves
      - Some young people need to show they are brave and courageous to enhance the self-esteem. They need to understand that being responsible is a way of being brave and courageous.
   2) What dificulties might you have if you support healthy behaviours?
      - Others might put you down or not agree with you
      - You might be laughed at
      - You might be excluded from the group.
   3) How might you overcome these problems?

Take a good risk. Stand up for healthy behaviours. Realize that you are helping ar supporting others, maybe even saving a life.

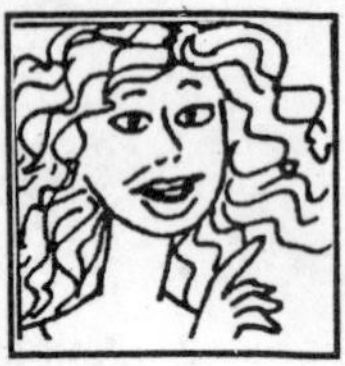

What the peer leader(s) does:

Peer leaders can:

- Act as a model for positive support in the classroom
- Be in charge of a small group
- Volunteer answers
- Read situations to students.

4.9. COMPASSLON, TOLERANCE AND SUPPORT

Purpose

Compassion, tolerance and support mean little to young people unless they are given the opportunity to actually practise these behaviours in everyday situations.

What the teacher does

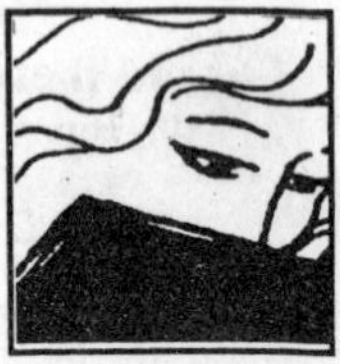

1. Read the list "Am I really compassionate?", to the students. Ask if they have other suggestions and add these to the list.
2. Have the students choose one from the list or make up one of their own.
   Then have them fill out their "Action plan" (sections 1, 2 and 3; section 4 will be completed after the action plan is carried out).
3. Set a date (two weeks will probably be enough) for completing the action plan and reporting back, in section 4, "Summary of what happened and my feelings". This section might include: how I felt; how the person I helped felt; what I did; how I did it; did it feel artificial or real - why; would I do it again; were there things I would do differently, etc.
4. Collect the summaries when finished and check to see that they were completed. Invite the students to discuss their experiences in class.

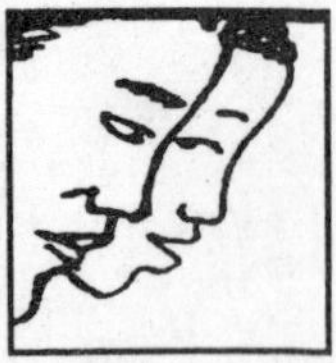

What the teacher does

Teachers should work with peer leaders to develop their action plan before the class so that these plans can be used as an example.

•••